MW01202129

An Intelligent Person's
Guide to Medicine

An Intelligent Person's Guide to Medicine

Theodore Dalrymple

Duckworth

First published in 2001 by
Gerald Duckworth & Co. Ltd.
61 Frith Street
London W1D 3JL
Tel: 020 7434 4242
Fax: 020 7434 4420
Email: enquiries@duckworth-publishers.co.uk
www.ducknet.co.uk

A catalogue record for this book is available
from the British Library

ISBN 0 7156 2973 5

Typeset by
Derek Doyle & Associates, Liverpool
Printed in Great Britain by
Biddles Limited, *www.biddles.co.uk*

The truth is not for all occasions.
Goldberg, A. 3. August 2009

Contents

1

Secular Salvation: Defining Health

The facetious Pontius Pilate demanded a definition of truth, but if he were alive today he would almost certainly ask instead for a definition of health: for people nowadays are much more concerned with their health than with truth.

Of course, the question 'What is health?' is no easier to answer than the question 'What is truth?' Down the ages, it has probably received at least as many answers, though most of us feel that we have an instinctive grasp of the meaning of both words. Health is thus a little like poetry: it is easier to say what it isn't than to say what it is.

According to the father of medicine, Hippocrates, health is that state of the human body in which the four constituent humours – that is to say, the blood, the yellow bile, the black bile and the phlegm – are in perfect harmony, with none in excess. But since we can only know that none of the four hypothetical humours is in excess by the presence of good health, Hippocrates doesn't get us very far. His definition is circular, though venerable and long lasting in its medical and literary influence. The poet Robert Herrick, about two thousand years later, wrote:

> Health is no other (as the learned hold)
> But a just measure both of Heat and Cold.

And more than three hundred years after Herrick, the definition of health was still unclear. The founding charter of the World Health Organisation, drawn up in 1946, stated grandiloquently that health was not the mere absence of disease, but the positive presence of physical, psychological and social wellbeing: health thereby becoming the summation of all other human desiderata. Henceforth, if the WHO was to be believed, everything under the sun was a matter of health – from a marital argument, for example, to the level of remuneration of postmen – and presumably doctors, as the guardians of health, were to become the universal busybodies. Only aspiring totalitarian dictators could have taken this definition seriously.

For Rousseau, health was the natural condition of Man which civilisation had subverted. The children of our ancestors, the noble savages, 'coming into the world with the excellent constitution of their parents, and strengthening it by the same means by which it was first produced, attained the full vigour of which the human species is capable.' From there, of course, it was downhill all the way:

> The extreme inequality in our way of life, the excessive leisure of some, the excessive work of others, the ease of exciting and satisfying our appetites and desire for sensual pleasure, the too-refined food of the rich, which stimulates their gastric juices and strikes them down with indigestion, the bad food of the poor, in insufficient quantities, whose very insufficiency causes them to overeat when the opportunity arises, the late nights, the excesses of every kind, the transports of all kinds of emotion, the fatigues, and the exhaustion of the spirit, the sorrows, and the innumerable hardships ... by which every soul is unendingly gnawed; there you have the sad proof that the majority of our illnesses are of our own making, and that we should have avoided almost all of them had we preserved the simple, steady and solitary way of life prescribed by Nature.

There is clearly a similarity between the views of Rousseau and Mary Baker Eddy, the founder of Christian Science, who regarded illness as theological error. Live either as nature or as God intended, and all will be well with you. But at the time in which he wrote, Rousseau's view was somewhat less absurd than it seems (or ought to seem) to us today. His view was shared by one of the great medical benefactors of Mankind,

Edward Jenner, who publicised, if he did not quite discover, vaccination against smallpox, and who wrote, 'The deviation of Man from the state in which he was originally placed by Nature seems to have proved to him a prolific source of disease.' Neither Rousseau nor Jenner could have known that a demographic revolution was about to take place, at the end of which the biblical span was an unduly conservative estimate for the life expectancy of hundreds of millions of people. Rousseau was expressing a mere prejudice rather than the result of deep research or even thought, but he was in a sense right: people in hunter-gatherer societies such as corresponded to his 'natural' state of Man probably did live longer and healthier lives – on average – than people in eighteenth-century France. That is to say, their life expectancy was probably forty years compared with thirty: though it is unlikely that any of them lived as long as it was possible for at least some people to live in conditions of civilisation even in Rousseau's day. Be that as it may, from the standpoint of the beginning of the third millennium, no population with a life expectancy of forty years could be considered healthy, and only the very poorest countries of Africa, with raging epidemics of AIDS and tuberculosis, have life expectancies anything as low as that of Rousseau's natural man.

Jeremy Bentham, the utilitarian philosopher whose mummified corpse sits in University College, London, in defiance (it seems to me) of his own utilitarian principles, defined health in his *Principles of Morals and Legislation* more modestly, with dry and pedantic caution, and therefore somewhat more usefully. Health is, according to Bentham, 'the absence of disease, and consequently of all those kinds of pain which are among the symptoms of disease. A man may be said to be in a state of health when he is not conscious of any uneasy sensations, the primary seat of which can be perceived to be anywhere in his body.'

This relatively sensible definition is not without its own problems, however. Let us lay aside for a moment the deliberate obfuscations of medical sociologists, who argue that disease is essentially a social construct, in proof of which they often cite a tribe of South American Indians among whom a certain fungal infection of the skin is so prevalent that they – the Indians – consider its absence rather than its presence to be the diseased state. This perverse view is only possible for professional, or academic, nit-pickers, with slight or intermittent contact with the realities that govern human life. But there are nevertheless other difficulties with Bentham's definition.

I would consider myself to be healthy, for example. But from time to time I am aware of a slight discomfort in one of my knees, the result of an injury in Africa many years ago. I am told that the injury will inevitably progress to osteoarthritis of the knee. Am I healthy when I do not feel the ache in my knee, but unhealthy when I do? This would seem to be the absurd consequence of Bentham's definition.

Osteoarthritis is not a life-threatening condition, of course, except perhaps on the savannahs of East Africa where Man is said to have evolved. My knee injury does not debilitate me or prevent me from doing much that I would have done without it, and unlike my African forebears I have no need to evade sabre-tooth tigers. So Bentham's definition might be saved by adding that the uneasy sensations of which a man in a state of health must be unaware should be those that are the consequence of a serious, debilitating or life-threatening condition. The thousand natural twinges that flesh is heir to do not count.

But even with this qualification, the definition has its difficulties. Suppose – as is not by any means unlikely – that somewhere within my entrails a cancer is growing. I am not aware of it, of course: most cancers have been present for several years before they make their unlucky host aware of their presence. I may feel in perfect health, but I am living in a fool's paradise. It is upon this fact (or rather, upon the fear of it) that the medical check-up industry depends, for no one can ever be quite sure that he is not incubating fatality within him. As usual, Shakespeare knew it:

> For within the hollow crown
> That rounds the mortal temples of a king
> Keeps Death his court, and there the antic sits
> Scoffing his state and grinning at his pomp,
> Allowing him a breath, a little scene
> To monarchise, be feared and kill with looks,
> Infusing him with self and vain conceit
> As if this flesh which walls about our life
> Were brass impregnable, and humoured thus
> Comes at the last and with a little pin
> Bores through the wall and farewell king!

When it comes to our health, we are all ultimately as vulnerable as Richard II.

High blood pressure is another symptomless disease, which predisposes both to strokes and heart attacks. Before the latter events supervene, the patient is aware of no symptoms, at least until the diagnosis is made, whereupon he might develop headaches or lassitude, or side effects if treatment is instigated. Symptoms in this instance follow diagnosis, not diagnosis symptoms. A controversy once raged as to whether high blood pressure could truly be considered a disease at all: with Lord Platt on one side arguing that those with high blood pressure were a distinct and abnormal population, and therefore that high blood pressure was a disease like any other, and Sir George Pickering arguing on the other side that people with high blood pressure were merely at the extreme end of a normal variation, and no more suffered from a distinct disease than, say, people who were abnormally tall. From the point of view of an individual person's health, however, the dispute was arcane, and brings to mind Hogarth's famous print of the squabbling uroscopists, those eighteenth-century pseudo-learned quacks who claimed they could diagnose every ill from inspection of the urine alone. Whether high blood pressure is disease or a normal variation, whether Platt or Pickering was right, the fact is that its consequences for the patient are the same.

Is a person who feels perfectly well but has dangerously high blood pressure (we often say 'suffers from', though he suffers nothing at all – at least until he is told that he is supposed to be suffering) healthy or not? He has an increased risk of contracting at least one of two life-threatening conditions, but he is statistically more likely than not never to suffer from either of them.

And who is to decide, then, whether a person is healthy: the doctor or the person himself? When Bentham speaks of 'the primary seat of [the uneasy sensations that] can be perceived to be anywhere in [the] body', he wisely leaves unanswered the question of who is to do the perceiving. Medical sociologists are inclined on this matter to side with Humpty Dumpty: 'The question is, which is to be master – that's all.' On this view, doctors merely serve their own interests, both individually and as a profession, when they claim special insight into a person's state of health. The doctor is engaged in nothing but a power struggle with the patient when he examines him for those occult diseases that have as yet given rise to no symptoms. He is merely establishing his power over the patient and thereby preserving his income. This explains the paradox that, as everyone (in aggregate) gets healthier, doctors are busier than ever. They have invented new terrors with which to assert their authority, maintain their standing and preserve their income.

This view is too categorical and too crude. Let us consider four possibilities (themselves oversimplified):

(i)   the person feels well and is well
(ii) the person feels well but is ill
(iii) the person feels ill but is well
(iv) the person feels ill and is ill

No one would dispute that the person in situation (i) is healthy – at least, he is as healthy as it is possible for a mere mortal to be. The view that life is an incurable disease, and that every moment lived is a moment nearer death, and is therefore in reality a moment of illness, is a poetical trope with a long history, but of no medical value. As Donne says:

> There is no health: Physitians say that wee
> At best, enjoy but a neutralitie.

And Tennyson says the same two and a half centuries later:

> Dust are our frames: and, gilded dust, our pride
> Looks only for a moment whole and sound;
> Like that long-buried body of the king,
> Found lying with his urns and ornaments,
> Which at a touch of light, an air of heaven,
> Slipt into ashes and was found no more.

Such an absolutist view is an implicit demand that our lives should be judged by an impossible standard, that of changlessness, eternal youth and immortality. (The great French physiologist Claude Bernard said that healthy people were sick people who didn't know it.) Of course, modern man – deprived of the religious hope of eternal life hereafter – increasingly does judge his life from this impossible standpoint, and makes himself unnecessarily miserable in the process: but our conception of health cannot, or at least should not, be determined by utopian dreams. The impossible has always been the enemy of the possible.

The person in situation (ii) is fortunate, perhaps – provided his feeling of wellbeing does not prevent him from seeking life-saving treatment until it is too late – but not healthy. The person in situation (iii) would once have been called healthy but hypochondriacal, though with the constant expansion (or should I say inflation?) of psychiatric diagnoses to cover every conceivable undesired or undesirable type of human behaviour or belief, a person who thinks that he is ill when he is not is now regarded as being in fact ill: that is to say, he is right about not being well, but is mistaken as to the nature and source of his illness. In short, you are ill if you think you are.

Nor is this all: to be ill in this modern fashion, a patient no longer has to be sincerely mistaken as to his state of health, but can lie about it consciously and still be considered ill, provided only that he lies consistently enough, and behaves as if he believes his lies to be truths. Thus a man who goes from hospital to hospital, faking symptoms – usually of a kind which, if present, would indicate serious disease, but whose physiological basis is impossible to disprove without elaborate and expensive testing – is said to suffer from a bona fide disease, namely Factitious Disorder. This fell disease consists (according to the *Diagnostic and Statistical Manual of the American Psychiatric Association*, third revised edition) of the intentional feigning of physical symptoms and a need to assume the sick role without any obvious motive other than to be treated by others as ill. But if to lie about your health is to be ill, then to boast about your bank account is to be rich.

No one, presumably, would dispute that the person in situation (iv) is in a poor state of health.

Good health is more like a gestalt than a scientific term with a clear definition. Everyone appreciates that good health is to an extent relative: that, for example, a healthy ninety-year-old cannot be expected to do at all that a healthy twenty-year-old can do with ease. Everyone understands that for someone to be in good health, a complete absence of pathology is not required: a man with a club-foot can be healthy. But if there is a relative component to our gestalt of health, there is an absolute component too: at no time or stage of life can a man be accounted healthy if he is riddled with malignant secondaries.

In actual practice, a new arbiter of a person's health has entered the field: the government. It used to be the case that a patient would go to his doctor when he felt unwell, hoping for cure, alleviation or at the very least for comfort and consolation. He believed that bad health invariably made itself manifest in symptoms; and the doctor agreed with him, and simply waited for patients to turn up.

Then, with the expansion of medical knowledge and technology, the doctor would take advantage of a patient's presence to test him for common conditions that he might have in incipient form without knowing it. His urine would be tested for glucose, indicative of diabetes; his blood pressure would be taken to exclude hypertension. It was the doctor who, on the basis of his personal understanding of his duty to his patients, undertook these tests.

Increasingly, however, the doctor is not the agent of his individual patient, but of the third party that pays for his patient's healthcare: that is to say of the state in state-run systems, and of insurance companies in private insurance-based systems.

Health is now virtually an actuarial concept, the doctor's role being to bring his patient into conformity with the notional person that statistical tables have demonstrated is the healthiest and longest lived. The patient should therefore be a certain weight, with a certain blood pressure and a certain level of cholesterol in his blood (the exact figure to be desired remaining a matter of dispute). He should consume certain foods and not others; he should adopt a certain lifestyle and avoid others; he should avoid certain habits as our forebears fled the plague (if they were able). Call no man healthy till he obeys all the latest instructions issuing from the government or insurance companies. As T.S. Eliot put it:

> We're all of us ill in one way or another:
> We call it health when we find no symptom
> Of illness.

Which is why, of course, we need endless check-ups. If we can't find the illness from which we are suffering today, perhaps another examination tomorrow will reveal it.

Good health is, of course, desirable: self-evidently so. No one would prefer ill health to good health, not even a hypochondriac. The hypochondriac, who appears to love his symptoms as others love their old friends, does not want to be truly ill: he wants instead all the privileges that are usually granted to the ill, who are excused routine and tedious duties, indulged in their eccentricities, and granted a sympathy that is frequently withheld from others, all without the inconvenience of genuine or incapacitating illness. One of the parties to the dispute about hypertension, Sir George Pickering, also wrote a book in which he alleged that the chronic illnesses of such eminent Victorians as Charles Darwin and Florence Nightingale were in fact elaborate ploys to avoid the social and domestic distractions that would have made their great work impossible. Their imagined illnesses allowed them to concentrate on it to the exclusion of all else.

Not surprisingly, good health has been extolled and apostrophised ever since the dawn of literature. Hippocrates said that a wise man ought to realise that health was his most valuable possession. Martial said that life was not living, but living in health. Rabelais said that, without health, life was but an image of death. Montaigne said that health was the only thing deserving that we employ time, sweat, trouble, worldly goods and even life itself in its pursuit: for without it, life was painful and oppressive. Ben Jonson was eloquent on the subject:

> O health! health! the blessing of the rich! the riches
> of the poor! Who can buy thee at too deare a rate,
> since there is no enjoying this world, without thee?

Webster agreed, saying that gold that buys health can never be ill spent. Descartes, in his *Discourse on Method*, said that health was, without doubt, the first and fundamental blessing of life.

Over and over again the same sentiments are uttered. John Gay, author of *The Beggar's Opera*, wrote:

Nor love, nor honour, wealth nor power,
Can give the heart a cheerful hour,
When health is lost.

James Thomson wrote that health is the principle of bliss, Laurence Sterne that he who has health has little more to wish for, and Thomas Jefferson that health was the first requisite after morality and worth more than learning. Thomas Carlyle said that health alone was victory, and Ralph Waldo Emerson that if he were given health and a day, he would make all the pomp of emperors ridiculous.

They were all mistaken. Of course, there are illnesses or degrees of illness that do render life a burden, so that death seems a more desirable alternative. But it is simply not true that ill health by itself necessarily renders life intolerable or meaningless: and if this is so, then good health cannot be an end in itself. We do not participate in the world that we may hope to enjoy good health: we hope to enjoy good health that we may participate in the world.

No one, for example, would call Stephen Hawking a man in the peak of health; but equally, no one would (I assume) argue that his life was therefore not worth living. Indeed, a case could be made for saying that it is Man's mortality, and illness as a constant reminder of that mortality, which spurs him on to his greatest achievements. Men who thought they had ten billion years of life ahead of them might indefinitely postpone their efforts on the grounds that tomorrow and tomorrow and tomorrow were other days. It is certainly not difficult to find in history examples of men who suffered ill health and yet created: and creation is an implicit affirmation of the worth of life.

Indeed, if ill health were necessarily the catastrophe that it is often assumed to be, the survival of the human species itself would be something of a mystery. For most of humanity's history, it has lived in abject ill health, certainly by comparison with our current standards of well being. But it is well within the capacity of the human race, thanks to its ability to reflect consciously on its own existence, to decline to reproduce itself: indeed, it is said that the Caribs and the Amerindians decided not to have children after the Spanish conquest, so unbearable had life become for them. The fact that men and women down the centuries thought the continuation of human life worthwhile, despite the prevalence – indeed, utter inescapability – of ill health, suggests that good health is not a precondition of a desirable or a desired existence.

The health conditions in which our ancestors lived were truly appalling. The lifetime chance of a woman dying in childbirth in Elizabethan England was about one in twelve. In Georgian London, a half of all children died before they were five years old. And yet neither the art nor the literature of those eras suggests that contemporaries found life intolerable. On the contrary, literary expressions of existential despair continue to grow ever more strident (though not necessarily more sincere) as health conditions improve. It is as if Mankind, having been granted more than the biblical span, did not really know what to do with it: for it is security which forces us to look into the abyss of meaninglessness. When life hangs by a thread, no one questions its value.

It is characteristic of most of Mankind, alas, that it appreciates what it has only when deprived of it. Freedom is most keenly appreciated (and often used best) by those who have known tyranny. 'The feeling of health,' said Georg Christoph Lichtenberg, 'is acquired only through sickness.'

At the same time, the well are inclined to imagine illness in catastrophic terms, and to exaggerate the extent to which it destroys the value of life. Even the process of normal ageing is regarded with horror by the young. I can remember thinking as a man in my early twenties that baldness was a state so unutterably horrible that death itself was preferable: for baldness represented lack of vigour, loss of attractiveness, extreme old age and even defeat by life. Oddly enough, as I began to lose my hair, I found that it mattered far less than I had thought, and that my mental powers were undiminished by the exposure of my scalp to the elements. I had been overhasty in my judgement, and I doubt that I am the only person ever to have made this mistake.

It is very difficult to guess in advance how we would react to certain experiences. Many people have wondered, for example, how they would conduct themselves under a totalitarian regime that rewarded behaviour that in other circumstances would be regarded as extremely criminal or morally reprehensible. The extent to which the German and French populations informed upon their neighbours must give us pause, before we declare with conviction that we would be moral heroes in similar circumstances.

When, therefore, we say that 'I would rather be dead than...', this is not so much the assertion of a literal truth as an expression of an emotional stance towards whatever it is that we say we should rather be dead than. Thus 'I had rather be dead than bald' means, in effect, 'I very much hope that I shall not lose my hair', and is certainly not an open invitation to Dr Kevorkian to put me down with his Mercitron as soon as a bald patch in my hair first becomes visible to others.

Most people would assume that life as a quadriplegic, paralysed from the neck down, is not worth living. The right of such a person to die was the subject of a successful play, *Whose Life Is It, Anyway?*, in which it was suggested that the medical and nursing staff who were trying to keep such a man alive against his will were acting unethically. Everyone should be allowed to die if he wants to.

In actual practice, however, quadriplegics do not want to die. They want to live. It is part of the glorious adaptability of Man that he can extract meaning and value from situations that seem unenviable. Even people who would have said before they became quadriplegic that, if ever they did so, they would not wish to continue to live find that, once it has happened to them, their attitude changes, and life seems more valuable to them than ever. Saying 'I would rather be dead than...' is characteristic of those in good health who have rarely experienced its opposite. The case of the quadriplegics who unexpectedly wish still to live illustrates the dangers of the living will. The limitations of the human imagination in comprehending what a hypothetical future state would be like make it dangerous to pronounce too rigidly about whether one could bear it or not.

This is not to say that there is no state of illness that renders the continuation of life a torment rather than a blessing. It is, however, to say that health is most definitely not a precondition of a worthwhile existence. I learned this lesson early in my life, since my best friend up to the age of eleven was a boy who contracted polio at the age of five which paralysed him from the waist down. He was fortunate, perhaps, in having a mother who was a Christian Scientist, who did not really believe in illness as commonly conceived. At any rate, she granted him no indulgence on the grounds of his disability, with the result that he went on to have a distinguished career in a field that one might have supposed would be closed to him. Certainly, there was never a suggestion that his tragic illness had deprived his life of all meaning and that it would have been better had he died (as some in those days still did) during its acute phase. While no one, surely, would argue that his illness was anything other than most unfortunate, no one would argue either that, because it deprived him of the ability to do many things that other boys could do, the value of his entire life was vitiated.

Another of my close friends at school during childhood had very severe asthma. It deformed his chest, and he also had generalised eczema that gave rise to scaling of his skin. He could play no games, and I remember still his laboured walking up the slightest incline, clutching his inhaler and stopping every few yards to take a puff at it. Despite the fact that the carefree physical pleasures of childhood could scarcely be his – he never kicked or hit a ball, for instance – he was not in the slightest sorry for himself, at least not in public. He asked for, and was given, no special sympathy. Although he had frequently to go to hospital because of crises in his condition, he never expressed the thought that life was not worth continuing. In fact, he believed that he had a brilliant future, for he was a gifted linguist with a precocious appreciation of literature. He was both serious and light-hearted. The fact that he had asthma to an exceptionally serious degree did not reduce his appetite for life, though of the reality of his suffering there could be no doubt.

Alas, his life was to be very short. One day, having been away for a week, I went to his house to see him. His mother opened the door to me: she was red-eyed with grief. He had died a few days before during one of his attacks. While she tried to summon an ambulance (she was believed at first to be exaggerating the seriousness of her son's condition, which led to a delay while the ambulance service verified his diagnosis with his general practitioner), he cried out, 'I'm dying, I'm dying!' He died just before the ambulance arrived. He was sixteen.

I have little doubt that, had he survived, his life would have been one of much suffering. I also have little doubt that it would have been one of much achievement and pleasure. It would have been better had he lived, suffered and achieved. His death was a tragedy. His exclamation that he was dying indicated that he wanted to live, though he could hardly have had many illusions as to his future state of health, and the problems to which it would have given rise, had he done so. He would have missed many of the normal gratifications of life, and yet he would have derived worth from his existence. Illness did not mean his life was not worth living.

The neurologist Oliver Sacks has written many startling case histories of people who, overtaken by what at first seem disastrous conditions, find a way of turning them to account: for example, of an artist who loses all colour vision and henceforth sees the world monochromatically. According to Sacks, his art subsequently widened and deepened in emotional range, though of course he went through a period of despair.

No binding rule can be laid down concerning the point at which illness deprives life of its worth. To try to lay down such a rule is to ignore one of the defining characteristics of human life, namely its reflexive nature. In general, the poorer the life before a disabling or incapacitating illness was contracted, the sooner that point is reached at which life is no longer considered worth living (though even so, one must not disregard the powerful imperative to survive at whatever expense of spirit). By contrast, the richer the life lived, the more suffering and debilitation that can be withstood without the supervention of a death wish.

Good health is not therefore the *summum bonum* of human existence, or the precondition of a worthwhile life, but merely one good among many. No one would prefer to be unhealthy than healthy, or at least to suffer the kind of ill health that might lead to a shortening of life; but a person who regarded as intolerable the slightest decline from the peak of health would be unbalanced, as unbalanced as someone who thought his life unlivable unless he were among the richest people in the world. People who pursue their health for its own sake – except in moderation and with the exercise not of muscles but of judgement – are rather like the hi-fi enthusiasts who used to devote themselves to the technical specifications of their apparatus, but never actually listened to music.

And yet there is little doubt that the promotion of health is now regarded as among the most important tasks of human life, or even as the task that surpasses all the others in importance. When something is bad for health, its prohibition requires no further philosophical justification. When something is good for health (more often notionally so than in reality, for it is easier to discover what is harmful than what is beneficial), its consumption or promotion likewise requires no further philosophical justification. Arguing against the all-importance of health in the current climate of opinion, however, is likely to draw strange looks. Is not the all-importance of health self-evident: more self-evident, indeed, than the truths of the American Declaration of Independence?

For the individual, healthiness is not next to godliness: it has replaced godliness. Doing what is (allegedly) good for one's health is the nearest anyone is allowed to come to virtue in an age that has lost faith in the traditional virtues. Practically no candidate for the presidency of the United States can escape the necessity of being photographed while out jogging: he plays the athlete as Marie Antoinette played the shepherdess. Joggers frequently have the expression on their faces that I imagine the flagellants of medieval times must have had: they are purging the sins of the world by their activity.

Recently I met a complacent jogger in his middle fifties who told me that he ran three hours every day and that he had never had a day's illness in his life: by which he meant, of course, that he had never had a day's illness in his life because he ran three hours a day. Only a saved, born-again Christian could have equalled him for moral complacency.

I pointed out to him that he was wasting approximately a fifth of his waking adult existence on his pursuit of health through running, and that, if he lived to be seventy, he would have spent ten years pounding the ugly pavements of the city. Why not just call it quits, and die ten years sooner? In fact, he had concluded a far worse bargain than that: and the deleterious effects on his prematurely arthritic hip joints were the least of it. It was highly unlikely that he would get his ten years back in extra longevity: perhaps one year, if any at all, was more like it. Moreover, the time he spent on running was time spent in the full vigour of his life, while the extra years he gained, if any at all, were at the other end of life, when life tends to be least vigorous and creative. It would be difficult to imagine time worse spent than his on running.

Unless, that is, it were time spent at a fitness club in the city in which I write this, whose gymnasium has a large, long window that gives on to the street, through which the passer-by can witness scores of women pedalling furiously on wheel-less bicycles and walking with grim determination on treadmills that produce nothing except sweat. People pedalling and walking to nowhere: here indeed is Sisyphus made flesh.

By the same token, the pursuit of health has turned meals virtually into medical procedures. All flesh is grass, of course: from which it unfortunately follows that all cancer is also grass. And not only cancer, but all the other ailments to which flesh is heir. This being the case, the prudent person had better watch his diet pretty carefully, if he does not want to fall victim to what were once called the diseases of civilisation, but in truth would be more accurately called the diseases of failure to die at an earlier age, as most humans did for the major part of their recorded and unrecorded history.

Needless to say, it is not easy to decide what to eat and what to avoid. Science is not a body of settled doctrine, to guide us in the paths of nutritional wisdom once and for all; it is (at least with regard to the healthful diet) a series of temporary hypotheses that, as any assiduous reader of those publications for incipient hypochondriacs, our newspapers, will be able to tell you, change not by the decade but by the week.

The dose makes the poison, of course, so that it is possible, by suitable extrapolation, to prove that any substance whatever constitutes a terrible hazard for the health. You could crush both laboratory animals and humans to death with a sufficient weight of any medication whatever; there is nothing in the world that is safe at every possible level of consumption, ergo there is nothing safe.

For the searcher after nutritional safety, there is no trade-off between health benefits and health costs. Something is either safe *tout court* or dangerous *tout court*. The ingredients of meals are either deadly poison or the elixir of life. On more than one occasion I have seen people turn orange with the amount of carrots they have consumed or carrot juice they have drunk, on the grounds that if a small dose of carotene is good for you, then immensely larger doses must be immensely better for you. Indeed, I once saw a couple with an orange baby, upon whom they had projected their panacean fantasies.

Most people do not go as far as that couple, of course, but still they are tormented by the question of whether what they eat is slowly killing them. They feel that if they juggle the components of their diet sufficiently shrewdly, they will either escape death altogether or, if it comes to them, it will be in that pleasant form described in the writings of Lieh-Tzu, the Chinese sage of about 400 BC, who said that there was a golden age in which people never died before they were a hundred, and never aged nor fell sick either. Why, or of what, they should have died the sage does not make clear: death would presumably have been something like a premed, when the person about to be operated upon swims pleasantly into oblivion at the end of the anaesthetist's needle. 'Just a little prick, dear, and then you'll be dead.' We are back in the world of Dr Kevorkian and his Mercitron.

Every meal is composed of untold numbers of ingredients, in virtually infinite combinations. To assess the health implications of all the ingredients individually, let alone severally in their various combinations, as would have to be done for any scientifically meaningful conclusions to be drawn, is a task enormously too complicated ever to be undertaken. The science of a single meal would take many lifetimes to work out properly, and the results would be of exiguous value. For Man would still have to eat, if every last comestible on earth were a carcinogen. In other words, for a man who took nutrition seriously, choosing what to eat would become a choice between an infinite and dizzying number of evils. He would never be at ease at the dining table. Socrates said that the unexamined life was not worth living: but it is a far, far better life than that which is too minutely examined.

Besides, the assumption that ill health is the consequence of bad diet is a very doubtful one, though ancient in its provenance. The Hippocratic corpus contains a book on regimen; and both dietary moderation and a simple life have long been

advocated as the key to longevity, if not to immortality.
Nutrition (with a few exceptions) has been to medicine what
astrology was to astronomy, or alchemy to chemistry. It is true,
of course, that the discovery of vitamin deficiencies was a great
triumph of nutritional biochemistry, and that this discovery
changed the entire aspect of medicine, which at the time was so
flushed with the triumph of the new bacteriology that practically all human ills were attributed to infection, that is to say
to a microbiological presence rather than to a nutritional
absence, so that there had been claims of bacterial causation
for vitamin deficiencies such as beriberi and pellagra; but just
as the germ theory of disease soon produced its fanatics who
wanted to wipe bacteria off the face of the earth in the name of
health-preserving cleanliness, so the discovery of vitamin deficiency gave rise to the general idea, still much in vogue, that
we are all, in some subtle way or another, suffering from one
nutritional shortage or other. One of the banes of my life as a
child (there were many, it goes without saying) was cod liver
oil, which came in little translucent brown rugby-ball-shaped
capsules that were fascinating to look at and squeeze, but
revolting to take: for though they tasted of nothing as you
swallowed them, a little while later fishy eructations from the
stomach occurred, like bubbles of poison gas emerging from
molten lava. The government of the time had decided –
wrongly, as it turned out, as it usually does turn out – that
British children were in imminent danger of Vitamin D deficiency, and so tens of thousands of squalling children were
cajoled, threatened and no doubt beaten into swallowing the
poison-gas capsules, so that the national shame of a child with
rickets might be avoided.

Of course, for every substance we lack that would do us
good, we consume a million that (allegedly) do us harm. Our
arteries are clogged up by food, our bowels are provoked into
cancerous growth by food, and – increasingly – we are allergic
to food. And there is scarcely an undesirable behavioural trait
that has not been attributed to a reaction to a previously

innocuous, but now poisonous, substance such as sugar: for example, it has been claimed in all seriousness, in a court of law, that it wasn't the killer who killed her, but the sugar he ate before he did so. And earlier in the week in which I write this, I heard of a boy aged fifteen who, according to his relative, had been diagnosed with the fell condition, Oppositional Defiance Disorder (that is to say he was bad tempered, disobedient and violent), an illness supposedly caused by the impurities of modern food, the precise culprit having yet to be named and shamed by the tedious process of elimination diets.

As to food allergies, everyone has them these days, or knows someone who has (a fifth of the British population claims to suffer from them, a proportion that is likely to grow with ever-wider publicity). It is likely that the real incidence has increased greatly of late, as has the incidence of asthma, one explanation being that an excess of public hygiene has deprived the immune systems of the young of real invasive enemies to fight and guard against. But perhaps even more noteworthy is that the number of people claiming to suffer from food allergies exceeds by a factor of at least ten the number who can be proved by objective tests to do so. It appears, then, that a large number of people want either themselves to suffer from, or their children to suffer from, food allergies.

Attitudes to ill health have sometimes been more ambiguous than you might suppose from all the grandiloquent apostrophising of robust good health that I have quoted above. Some illnesses have at certain epochs been fashionable, for example gout in the eighteenth century. To have gout was then regarded as a sign that one belonged to, or had joined, polite society: for it had been noticed that gout more frequently struck the wealthy and the educated than the poor and the ignorant. The gouty lived longer than the great mass of the non-gouty, and so it was quite reasonably (though nonetheless erroneously) concluded that gout was not only a sign of high social standing, but was actually good for you: that, rather like the laudable pus of later surgical theorising, it represented the vigorous expulsion of harmful matter from the body. Thus men who became gouty were often pleased by it because, painful as were the symptoms, they saw in it a guarantor of their own longevity.

In fact, people with gout lived longer because they were richer, not because they were gouty; and rich people live longer than poor people (with one or two notable exceptions). Yet the good reputation of gout as an illness lived on well into the twentieth century, and when my father first contracted it, with an inflammation of his big toe so exquisitely painful that any movement of the air in his bedroom was intolerable to him, I had little difficulty in finding statements in medical textbooks regarding what financiers would call the upside of the disease: that gout rarely subsisted with coronary artery disease and that it was more common among the highly intelligent.

Food allergies are, in some ways at least, the modern equivalent of gout: or perhaps of tuberculosis, as portrayed in romantic literature and opera. Such allergies do not, of course, stand guarantor of longevity: but they are in their own way a sign of the elect. It is precisely the rarity (though slight possibility) of a fatal outcome which is their attraction. Because of the obvious similarity of the words sensitivity and sensibility, people regard alleged food allergies as evidence that they are too finely wrought for this unfeeling world in which we unhappily find ourselves. Their bodies are able to make distinctions that grosser natures cannot make. Food allergy – of the alleged rather than the real variety, since the real is a real nuisance – is a form of modern dandyism, connoisseurship and aestheticism.

Of course, the belief in a hypersensitivity too subtle for the current methods of science to detect has more than one advantage. It suits the anti-authoritarian spirit of the age, and scientific medicine is one of the few authorities still sufficiently undamaged to be worth undermining. A negative is impossible to prove; it is always possible that future, hitherto undeveloped tests will show that the complainant was right all along; and the history of medicine is replete with error, both on matters of doctrine and in matters of individual diagnosis and treatment. There are more things in heaven and earth than are dreamed of in anyone's philosophy; and to prove doctors (or any other authorities) wrong is one of the few ways men and women in mass society can assert their individuality. To be a puzzle to conventional science (without, of course, true debilitation) is a fine boost to the ego, and an invaluable aid to self-importance.

Of course, the desire to be ill through sensitivity sets up its own competition: mirror, mirror on the wall, who's the most allergic of them all? The answer, it turns out, is the person who claims to be allergic to everything, or at least to everything that is produced industrially with the help of chemicals. Total chemical sensitivity has been called allergy to the twentieth century, or Twentieth-Century Disease, though I doubt that it ceased on the stroke of the midnight hour on 31 December 1999 (or 2000, if you want to be strictly accurate). Such people say they can live only in very special environments, coddling themselves and protecting themselves from the less attractive aspects of modern life. And I remember a woman who exported her sensitivity to a remote region in rural Africa, maintaining that there was only one particular brand of bottled water – from Germany – that she could drink and bathe in without ill effect. The cost of her little foible was astronomical.

Why should anyone want to be ill in this fashion? It is only an extreme form of modern hypochondriasis: for despite objective statistical evidence that people are healthier than ever before in the whole history of humanity, living on average three times as long as in the eighteenth century, surveys demonstrate that people have an intense dissatisfaction with their state of health, and worry more than ever about their present and future physical condition.

Illness or the threat of ill health automatically gives meaning and purpose to life, without further soul-searching. It provides a ready-made solution to the question of how one should spend one's life: one should spend it in pursuit of a cure or in the avoidance of the cause or causes of illness. The more difficult and philosophically embarrassing question of how best to live is thus indefinitely postponed.

The belief that health is the indispensable precondition of a worthwhile life, when taken seriously, exerts a corrosive effect upon the character. The preservation of health becomes a person's highest moral duty, a kind of hypochondriac's Kantian categorical imperative. It empties the world of true moral content: for every moral dilemma comes to be seen from the point of view of physical safety or the effect of the various possible courses of action upon the health of the person who is involved in the dilemma. A person who acts on the current received wisdom for the preservation of health feels morally superior to someone who wilfully fails to do so (such superiority is writ large on the faces of joggers). Correspondingly, those who like chocolate or don't like exercise are made to feel guilty, as if they were failing in their duty to themselves and to society: for if they become avoidably ill as a result of their own negligence, they will be a burden on others.

Safety is now a desideratum that trumps all others. If a course of action is deemed to increase safety – that is to say, the physical integrity of people – no further argument is required to demonstrate that it is the correct course of action. It is self-evidently correct.

I can give an example from my very doorstep. The area in which I live, and where I write this, is infested with prostitutes. They are brought in shifts from outlying areas on buses owned by pimps. The kerb-crawlers of the city need never go without relief of their overwhelming sexual desire, and I have noticed, when called out while on duty for my hospital, that even at eight o'clock on a Sunday morning prostitutes make themselves available on street corners. Some of them are clearly under age: no older than thirteen or fourteen.

The local health authority funds a large van that cruises the area, distributing condoms to the women and girls. This is to make their activities safer, so that they neither catch nor transmit venereal diseases, including, of course, AIDS. Whatever they do, they must do it safely: for safety is the highest aim in life.

That other public responses to child prostitution of this nature are possible seems not to have been considered, a fact that future historians might surely consider extremely odd, in view of the prevailing mass hysteria about paedophilia and the great public concern displayed about the sexual abuse of children. So great has been the reaction against Victorian moralism, indeed, that those who would once have patrolled the streets to redeem the fallen girls are now patrolling the streets to hand them condoms: the encouragement of their physical wellbeing (or at least the avoidance of illness) being the nearest to the promotion of virtue that anyone can nowadays attain without appearing judgemental. (In medical journals, it is now *de rigueur* to speak of prostitutes as sex workers and of prostitution as the sex industry: though pimps have yet to be renamed sex facilitators, sex promoters or sex impresarios.)

It might be, of course, that after careful consideration of all aspects of the problem, the distribution of free condoms would still be the policy best adopted. If, for example, it was proved with a fair degree of certainty that there must always be thirteen- or fourteen-year-old prostitutes on street corners, because it is an inevitable and ineradicable part of urban existence, and that all attempts to suppress such prostitution necessarily fail or are counterproductive, then obviously it would be better that thirteen- or fourteen-year-old prostitutes should neither catch nor spread venereal diseases. But I suspect that no serious attention was given to other methods of approaching the problem because their goal would not have been safety, the one good that transcends all other goods and the one purpose that unites all people of goodwill.

Similarly, it has been suggested in the prison in which I

work that there should be a needle exchange set up so that prisoners can inject themselves with heroin in comparative safety: at least from the risk of infecting themselves with the AIDS virus.

The reasoning behind the proposal is as follows. It is well known that many convicted criminals are heroin addicts, and that moreover heroin is available in prisons to those who want it. Some prisoners will continue to inject even in prison, and since it is the sharing of needles rather than the injecting per se which spreads the virus, giving prisoners easy access to clean needles whenever they wish to inject themselves will result in harm reduction, that is to say less illness and greater safety.

Proponents of this view sweep aside both the philosophical and practical objections to the proposal. It is, for example, no part of the prison's duty to save prisoners from the harmful consequences of their own illegal conduct. And there are other possible public responses to vice than to make it safe for those who practise it.

Moreover, the proposal ignores, as is so often the case, the reflexive nature of human behaviour. It is true that the spread of the virus is somewhat reduced in prisons in which there are needle exchange schemes; but it is also true that in prisons in which there are no needle exchange schemes the majority of those who would otherwise have continued to inject heroin stop doing so, precisely because they know the dangers. A minority continue in their habit and risk becoming infected; the majority do not.

This example also illustrates another aspect of risk that is often overlooked by the zealous proponents of a favoured form of risk reduction: that to reduce risk in one direction is often to increase it in another, since practically all forms of human conduct (both acts and omissions) entail risk. In the case of the proposed needle exchange scheme in prison, the number of prisoners contracting the AIDS virus might be reduced; but in so far as the needle exchange scheme would encourage people to continue to inject themselves with heroin, it would increase their risk of dying of an injected overdose.

Those who see the reduction of risk as being the be-all and end-all of policy would, of course, favour the adoption of the needle exchange scheme if it could be proved that the risk of contracting AIDS in the absence of the scheme were greater than the risk of dying of an overdose in its presence (something they would be inclined to believe, because activists always want to do something rather than nothing). But even if it were beyond doubt that needle exchange schemes in prisons did, on balance, save lives, it would still be possible to oppose them: provided it was accepted that safety is not the only aim of human life or public policy. Increasingly, though, this is difficult to argue: for safety is to the secular what salvation was to the religious.

Because safety guarantees health in the way that salvation once guaranteed eternal life, the person who adopts the latest allegedly healthful lifestyle does not consider himself merely prudent, but virtuous. A healthy lifestyle fills the gap in the moral economy where respectability used to be. Faith, hope and charity have been replaced by no smoking, no animal fat and exercise.

Those who deny themselves indulgences of the flesh for the sake of their health often react to the news that they are ill with the same illnesses from which the self-indulgent suffer with something approaching moral indignation. Why have they avoided butter, cream and cigars all these years if, in the end, it all comes to the same? They react much as I imagine a Puritan would react, who during his life never laughed or enjoyed himself, kept a sour expression, and strongly advocated the closure of theatres and all places of public entertainment, who found his soul after his death relegated to eternal hellfire, on the grounds that, actually, the Lord approved of singing and dancing and couldn't abide a killjoy. He wouldn't be very pleased.

In the countries of the north, where protestantism has

always made unselfconscious indulgence in pleasure psycho-logically problematical, if not impossible, certain aspects of hedonism become a medical duty rather than a natural way of life. Thus the exercise of uninhibited sexual freedom has been transformed into a right and a duty: which explains why there is little so unerotic as northern European pornography. This is because to indulge in previously forbidden sexual practices in public now has an almost evangelical quality to it: people display their virtue by breaking taboos. Many people have puzzled over why it should be that the advocates of the allegedly healthy lifestyle, who are so ascetic and thin-lipped in most regards, should be so indulgent with regard to sex, and insistent that something which is pleasurable is actually a good thing. The answer, as my friend Dr Digby Anderson has pointed out, lies in the fact that sexual activity involves exer-cise. We are told by the health zealots that we should set our hearts racing for a certain period of time every day, and of course sex does this better than anything else. Love is the extension of callisthenics by other means.

When it was discovered that alcohol in moderation – espe-cially red wine – was good for the health (or at least statistically associated with a slightly increased life expectancy, which is not quite the same thing), a spectre began to haunt the land: the compulsory medicinal glass of red wine for those who don't care for it. After all, if people who failed to take exer-cise were in part responsible for their illnesses, could it not henceforth be said that so, too, were teetotallers, in as much as refraining from drinking is at least as voluntary as drinking to excess? And the fact that many people who otherwise don't seem to know much now know the precise alcohol content of various drinks, as measured in 'units', as well as the recom-mended number of units to be consumed per week, suggests that the consumption of alcohol is well on the way to becoming medicalised. Just as some people go to the doctor's surgery to socialise, so people will soon be going to the pub for a little medicine.

It is very difficult to free oneself entirely from the modern obsession with health and safety as the measure of all things, even when, as in my case, one is philosophically opposed to it. For example, I cannot see a smoker without experiencing a frisson of puritanical disapproval and irritation. Does not the person realise the harm he is doing to himself with his habit? Hasn't he been told often enough of the dangers of smoking? And yet he persists!

Unlike so many epidemiological associations, of the kind that lead, on publication, to sudden gusts of public panic or over-optimism, the causative association between smoking and ill health seems to me to be well founded. Smoking is very bad for you (and is, moreover, aesthetically unpleasing to those who don't smoke, a fact that smokers have difficulty in believing, at least until they themselves give up smoking). Of course, every smoker has an uncle who smoked sixty cigarettes a day and lived to be ninety-eight: but the exhibition of such putative uncles as evidence for the harmlessness of smoking is a form of whistling in the wind. The evidence against smoking is conclusive.

Like the common-or-garden zealot, I am apt to forget that the harmfulness of tobacco to the health does not necessarily end the discussion: that there is more to be said. One of the first wards in which I worked as a clinical student was full of men with a rare disease of the arteries, found only in smokers. It led to the amputation of their limbs because of gangrene – first their legs and eventually, in some cases, their arms. They were told well in advance that if they continued to smoke they would most likely lose a further limb, but none of them stopped smoking. Even those with only one arm left – or neither – continued to smoke.

I was outraged. How could these men (they were all men) make so foolish a choice? The strength of their addiction did not answer the case: my own mother had given up smoking after twenty-five years, without apparent difficulty. She simply wanted to: and if her, why not them?

I asked them, with irritation gnawing at my young and intolerant vitals. They replied that they liked smoking, and that it was virtually the only pleasure they had left in life. Lady Bracknell, who approved of Ernest's smoking because she thought that a man should always have a hobby, would have applauded my patient who replied, when I asked what his interests were, 'Smoking.' And if a man is to be allowed to prefer, or perhaps even to be praised for preferring, the risks of mountaineering or polar exploration to the safety of a sedentary life, why should a man be criticised for preferring the pleasures of smoking to the benefits of abstention?

It might be answered that some risks are inherently more worth taking than others: that, for example, the mystical joy that a mountaineer feels on reaching an inaccessible peak is worth greatly more than the pleasure produced for the habitual smoker by a drag on a fag; but if so, the risk of ill health cannot be the measure of all things. Serious mountaineering is vastly more dangerous than smoking, as will readily be appreciated by imagining how many more would die prematurely if every smoker took to the Alps. Then indeed we should see premature death.

It is clear that the assessment of the significance of risk is a moral rather than a purely mathematical or technical one. I remember once reading a small item in the *British Medical Journal* not long ago to the effect that there were seventeen million sports injuries per year in Britain. There it was, this gigantic figure: no fuss at all. This, of course, was because sport was, *a priori*, a Good Thing, in the Sellar and Yeatman sense of the words. One has only to imagine the outcry there would have been had it been revealed that seventeen million people were injured while – or rather, because of – eating chocolate. Every confectioner in the country would have been arrested, lawsuits would have followed, and allegations of suppression of information made against the chocolate companies. The complete absence of comment on the figure published in the *BMJ*, either within or without the journal, establishes beyond reasonable doubt that the concerted outcry against tobacco is more in the nature of a moral crusade than a public health campaign. I should point out (before anyone makes a snide suggestion) that I have no shares in tobacco companies, and have never made a profit from cigarette sales: unlike, for example, the lawyers who have led the litigation in the United States against the tobacco companies, whose profits they have, in effect, transferred from the companies' shareholders to themselves. This, perhaps, explains why none of them, for all their forensic moral fervour, wishes to drive the companies into bankruptcy: for then there would be no one, or no one very lucrative, to sue.

I admit, however, that I retain the prim medical attitude to smoking. I cannot see a cigarette in the mouth of a patient without animadverting internally on his weakness of will, his lack of moral fibre, his complete stupidity – in short, his defective character. Moreover, as a doctor I conceive it my duty to advise my patients, in the strongest possible terms, not to smoke. The relatively small part of my make-up that is self-righteously sadistic even enjoys (until guilt at my own sadism supervenes) telling someone he must give up his cigarettes or die. When someone with a disease said to be more common in smokers tells me that he does not smoke I feel cheated of my prey.

And yet I admire people who disobey doctor's orders – provided their disobedience does not arise out of mulish refusal to believe the evidence. I once had a patient in a far-off land, a man of generous proportions, who consulted me about some swelling of his ankles. In the course of the consultation, he told me that he was diabetic.

I suspected that he was a bon viveur.

'You don't smoke, I suppose?' I asked, tentatively.

'Like a chimney,' he replied.

'Or drink?'

'Like a fish.'

By then, I had caught his drift.

'Of course, you love rich food?'

'I cook everything in cream and butter.'

I swiftly skated over the dangers of his mode of life. I told him nothing he did not already know. Nor did he deny that what I said was true. He simply said that he had considered the alternatives, and had decided to live as if his diabetes did not exist, except is so far as it was possible to keep his blood sugar level within normal limits by the use of medicine. There was a magnificence to his performance which I could not but admire, and we became fast friends. He had decided that the best was not necessarily the longest life, and – unlike so many – he had the courage of his convictions. He did indeed die earlier than he might have done, but I could not regard the loss of longevity as a waste of possible life.

Few have his courage: resistance to the medical view of existence is generally less conscious, or less honest. But still it does my heart good (I am talking of my metaphorical heart, of course) to see people *en masse* doing what the doctors say is bad for them. A few years ago, I visited a bingo club, to see what it was that so many of my older patients said they enjoyed. A doctor should know his patients, and that means when they let their hair down as well as when they are on their best behaviour, telling him that they put on weight though they hardly eat a thing.

The club was in a disused cinema. There were hundreds of people present, mainly past their fifties, fat, immobile, and drinking pints of beer while guzzling plates of greasy food and smoking like steam trains. There was a dense fug in the auditorium of the cinema, and the nearest any of the participants came to exercise, I should imagine, was waddling to the taxi that took them home afterwards. As a doctor I should have been appalled; but as a man, I was delighted. Here was innocent, convivial jollity: not my cup of tea as far as entertainment is concerned, but not the kind of purse-lipped parsimony that is enjoined by the health Pharisees, either.

For many, the pursuit of health, which is thought to require iron self-control over perfectly normal and harmless appetites, ends in precisely its opposite. Our obsession with the health-giving and health-sapping qualities of food has coincided with an enormous increase in the numbers of people who have difficulty in regulating what they eat, in the process either starving themselves half to death, or consuming gargantuan quantities of food well beyond the demands of hunger. Not since the health consequences of the contents of our diet became such a matter of obsessive interest – in the newspapers, on the radio and television, in daily conversation – have there been so many grossly fat or unhealthily thin people.

The quest for health is modern man's search for transcendence, and safety and danger are his good and evil. Good and evil embarrass him, whereas safety and danger are comfortingly naturalistic. No one can be against safety and in favour of danger. Allegedly the two can be quantified, though of course only a life of zero danger and perfect safety, in which there is no risk at all, is acceptable.

Modern man's concern with his health is a symptom – if I may use a medicalising metaphor – of his increasing solipsism. He is worried about himself and only himself. His solipsism is evident even when he gathers together in large numbers. His activities then are not so much social as atomistic. New forms of 'social' life, such as nightclubs in which thousands of young people gather, are in fact manifestations of mass solipsism: not only is dancing solitary and narcissistic, with each person performing in a kind of psychological capsule that excludes the presence of others, but the fundamental requirement of true social life, conversation, is impossible because of the noise.

Likewise, the concentration in our newspapers on matters of health (a recent phenomenon, as a perusal of the newspapers of even thirty years ago will attest) is simultaneously a manifestation of the rise of mass self-importance and of an involution of people's range of interest. Once upon a time people read newspapers in order to read about others; now they read them to read about themselves: for what are all the articles about health if not a form of self-absorption?

And this self-absorption exemplified by concern with matters of health and safety gives the government the *locus standi* to interfere with the most intimate details of our life: to issue advice and guidelines, pronounce norms, mandate tests, and turn doctors into mere functionaries of the state. Without our concern for health, indeed, the government would be much reduced in importance, since a consensus has been reached, except for minor details, over the way the economy should be run. Such consensus is incompatible with the rulers' self-image as saviours of their society: and no one devotes years of his life, perhaps even the whole of his life, to seeking office when office itself is of limited importance.

This is not to say that there are no matters which require and would be worthy of the attention of politicians. On the contrary: in Britain alone there is the matter of the general cultural and educational level of much of the population, in my experience (and I have worked and travelled in many parts of the world) the lowest not only in Europe, but in practically the entire world. The British educational system is, in much of the country, nothing but an expensive form of child neglect and abuse. Never in the field of human history has so little been taught to so many at such expense.

But the rectification of this situation would require real moral courage, the very quality most lacking among the place-seekers. Even the recognition of the problem – so obvious that it can be seen just walking down any English street – is beyond their level of courage. Instead, they seek non-problems to solve, concerning health: for everyone is agreed that health and safety come before all. A concentration on health is a way of averting the gaze from far graver problems afflicting society.

Recently, for example, the British minister of public health suggested that the children of today might not live as long as their parents because of their diet, which contains too little fruit and vegetables, and too much high-fat, salty and sugary food. There was not the faintest evidence for her assertion that the life expectancy of children was falling. All the indications are quite the reverse. In the United States, where the diet of junk food has been taken for longer, life expectancy has continued to increase. There are very few countries in the world where life expectancy has fallen instead of increased: Russia being notable among them, for its own special reasons, and the sub-Saharan countries of Africa, afflicted by the epidemic of AIDS, being the others. But the evidence is that diet affects life expectancy very little, unless it is grossly deficient in essential nutrients or in calorific quantity.

The minister, however, alluded to a very real problem, though in selecting its health consequences she displayed the miserable moral cowardice we have come to expect of our leaders. For the fact is that an increasing proportion of the population in Britain eat like asocial savages. A sociologist recently informed me that half the households in Britain no longer have a dining table, and whether this is true or not, I have observed that in most of the households into which I enter in the course of my medical duties, there is no evidence of real cooking (as compared to reheating industrially prepackaged meals) ever having gone on, or of meals taken in a social fashion around a table. By contrast, the ground outside such homes is strewn with the detritus of literally hundreds of meals bought from fast food chains and consumed on the street: for the Englishman's street is now his dining room.

It was once regarded (quite rightly) as uncouth and antisocial to eat in the street. What, then, does mass consumption of meals in the street signify, culturally speaking?

In the first place, it means that people are no longer able or willing (philosophers might dispute which) to ignore their appetites of the moment for the sake of social propriety and decorum. Their pangs of hunger can hardly be greater than those of their forebears: they are simply less tolerant of delayed gratification. And their snatching of something to eat, indiscriminately and undiscriminatingly, whenever and wherever they might be, indicates that they live in a fundamentally asocial, atomistic world, where families as anything other than temporary associations of human atoms scarcely exist: for there is no more fundamental social activity than eating together. To cook and eat well are beyond doubt social activities: which is why, for example, the Indians in the very same area in which there is so much feral asocial nourishment (where meals are nasty, solitary, British and short) eat properly, and why Indian housewives may still be seen choosing food carefully in grocers' shops, rather than shovelling it into a trolley as quickly as possible, to get the whole process over with as soon as possible. Whatever their problems, Indians tend still to eat meals together, for they do not yet live the atomised life of their native neighbours.

In other words, the public health minister was perfectly right to discern a problem in the diet of many British children, but her understanding of its significance was completely vitiated by the modern obsession with health and safety.

In summary, good health is obviously a desideratum of human existence, but it should not be valued for its own sake. It is neither a necessary nor a sufficient condition of a good life. An obsession with health is an inherently trivialising phenomenon, which obscures much more important aspects of life. No man should pursue good health except *grosso modo*, for example by immunising himself against serious infectious diseases that can be immunised against, or by taking prophylactics against malaria in malarious areas. Not every risk is worth avoiding, nor is every risk not worth taking. In our modern circumstances, the road to hell is paved with health.

2

Paying the Piper:
Delivering Healthcare

Healthcare is like government in Africa: no known system works. At least, no known system of healthcare works if it is judged by the standards of perfection or those of the ideal normal, according to which no problems are ever evident, no dissatisfaction ever arises, no mistakes are ever made, no waste ever occurs, and no one ever dies unnecessarily. Given the fallibility of Man, this is a completely useless standard by which to judge anything.

Viewed from another angle, all known systems of healthcare work: at least, those that exist in the Western world (which includes Japan). The indices of health in Western countries are more notable for their similarities than their differences: which suggests that their healthcare systems do not differ as much – at least in their effectiveness – as might at first sight be supposed. However different they may appear, all health-care systems do most of what they are supposed to do: or else healthcare is a relatively unimportant determinant of a nation's health.

Nevertheless, lively or even bitter controversies rage in most countries about their healthcare systems. This is for at least three reasons: first, Man is a squabbling animal; second, the grass is always greener on the other side (they order things better there); and third, present problems, however trifling in historical context, always loom larger in the mind than past accomplishments, however great.

Despite the fact that, whatever country one visits, people are always complaining, the illusion persists that, somewhere, the secret of a happy and harmonious existence has not only been discovered, but put into practice. As far as healthcare is concerned, this means a country in which arguments about funding never occur (everyone having agreed in advance that no sum is too great to secure so great an objective as the nation's health), in which the latest technology is instantly available to all who need it (the spread of medical technology to those who don't need it or who are harmed by it never happens in this medical Arcadia), and where consequently everyone lives to a ripe old age untroubled by serious or incurable illness. Needless to say, this happy state of affairs exists nowhere, has never existed anywhere, and never will exist anywhere: which is why it exerts so powerful a hold over the imagination.

We are not fully rational creatures, however: we can dream of and believe in the impossible, and grow angry over its non-fulfilment in reality. The eyes of faith are stronger than the mills of logic. In my small library, for example, I have several books about the miracles wrought by the Soviet healthcare system in the 1930s, written by doctors, not necessarily themselves communist sympathisers, who paid visits to model clinics (often in the midst of famine) and saw how the new government was defeating everything from TB to neurosis. When I was a medical student, the Chinese Cultural Revolution caught the imagination of a surprising number of my classmates, who at the time felt strongly the humiliation of being at the bottom of the medical hierarchy, and so found inspiration in the story of a Chinese peasant woman with an enormous ovarian tumour, which the doctors declared to be inoperable but for whose removal a hospital cleaner suggested a successful method. This feat of what was known at the time as Mao Tse-Tung Thought indicated that the way to medical salvation lay not through arduous and detailed technical researches, whose success could not be guaranteed in advance, but by the application of a few political precepts that were to

be found in the little plasticated red book of the Great
Helmsman and Oncologist. The destruction of the hierarchical
system under which medicine was practised was therefore the
indispensable condition by which the health of the population
was to be improved. Even today, in a pale reflection of those
utopian dreams, one sees medical study tours to China advertised in the pages of the medical journals, undertaken one
suspects not in the expectation of finding particular ameliora-
tions of particular diseases, but in the hope of finding a global
solution to all Man's medical problems.

The desire that all problems should be solved at once is, of
course, composed of laziness and impatience, with a leavening
– in some cases – of philanthropic sentimentality. That is why
the purveyors of panaceas never lack for customers, or indeed
are rarely themselves wholly without belief in their wares. In
the week in which I sat down to write this, for example, there
fell from my newspaper a little brochure advertising, with all
appearance of sincerity on the part of the promoter (a rene-
gade doctor), the stupendous healing powers of magnets. No
human ailment, it seemed, could resist the mysterious
magnetic efflux: nothing, from agoraphobia to haemorrhoids.
Since nothing is advertised – certainly on such a scale –
without the expectation of finding a buyer, and since it is prob-
able that the promoter did not believe himself to be an
unscrupulous scoundrel, it seems that a portion of humanity is
engaged upon a *pas de deux* between the purveyor and
consumer of nonsense. I mention this only as background:
there is no subject on which it is easier to fool some of the
people all of the time than that of health.

Even those who, influenced by rumours of the scientific
method, are disinclined to believe in the curative powers of
magnets are inclined to believe that somewhere there must be
a system of healthcare that reconciles all the various demands
that can be placed upon it: for speed, efficiency, humanity, flex-
ibility, comfort, economy, justice, equity, modernity and
infallibility.

Let us consider these many virtues individually and severally. It will be seen that they are not all compatible, and that it will, alas, sometimes be necessary to choose among them, according to priorities about which there are themselves intrinsically irreconcilable disputes.

First, however, we must bear in mind what is at stake: less than the passions evoked by the disputes might lead us to suppose. To recapitulate: first, health is not all important; second, it is not determined solely or even principally by the reigning system of healthcare; and third, all likely systems of healthcare do most of what they are supposed to do. Ordinary people would understand this better if it were not so much in the interests of politicians to magnify the scale of the problems and the likelihood of all-encompassing solutions, to magnify their power and self-importance. When people decide to leave one country for another, their choice of destination is little influenced by the kind of healthcare system they expect to find on arrival. For example, the system of healthcare in the United States is repeatedly excoriated (rightly or wrongly) for its failure to attend to the needs of precisely that stratum of society that immigrants are most likely to join: but this consideration does not in the least prevent the United States from being the most favoured destination of the world's poor.

Controversies over healthcare systems are therefore to an extent artificial, at least in their heat. They are a symptom of modern man's incessant need and insatiable appetite for public disputations, which are to him what gladiatorial combats were to the Roman mob, and which no doubt relieve his feelings of existential anxiety and emptiness. For modern man, the lack of a crisis is itself a crisis.

Nevertheless, there is little doubt that the healthcare systems of the world differ sufficiently to exercise the minds of almost everyone. This is because everyone can imagine himself ill and in need of treatment, because almost everyone either has been ill or will be ill: few are those who die in bed, never having previously known a moment's physical unease. And we all know how we should like to be treated when we are ill: expeditiously, effectively, humanely and comfortably – and, preferably, cheaply.

It is evident that economy and expedition are not entirely compatible. For everyone to be treated the moment he wishes – that is to say, the moment he is aware, or merely thinks, that he has a medical problem – there must be a large number of doctors and nurses in practice, and adequate facilities available. But demand has a way of expanding with supply, and some sorts of shortages always make themselves felt.

There are disadvantages, too, in immediate access to medical consultation and treatment. Most of the illnesses to which we are subject are self-limiting: that is to say, will go away of their own accord. If every time we feel a discomfort we fly to the doctor, we place ourselves in danger of being over-investigated and over-medicated. On the one hand, in a climate of increasing legal acrimony, doctors fear missing a diagnosis, however remote the chances of it being correct, by omitting to perform a test, even where the potential harms of the tests have a much greater statistical likelihood of occurring than any harm caused by the missed diagnosis. Moreover, it is possible for patients to become 'addicted' to unnecessary investigative procedures. On the other hand, doctors find it difficult to send patients away completely empty handed. Patients are likewise reluctant to abstain from taking medicine (the desire to do so being, according to the great turn-of-the-century physician Osler, one of the characteristics that distinguish Man from the animals), and regard doctors who prescribe nothing as mere ciphers, as whited sepulchres. I would be a rich man indeed if I had been financially rewarded each time I had had the following conversation:

'Have the pills helped you?'

'No.'

'Then I think we'd better stop them.'

'You can't do that, Doctor, how will I manage without them?'

The doctor prescribes, not only to treat the patient, but to treat himself. A prescription eases the patient out of the room, ending the consultation with what theorists of narrative are apt to call a satisfactory 'closure'. The doctor thinks he has done something for the patient, and the patient thinks the doctor has done something for him. Especially is this so for illnesses, or complaints, with a large psychological component; and all is well, at least until the patient begins to take the medicine prescribed.

Unhappily, doctors are not allowed any longer knowingly to prescribe placebos, that is to say physiologically inert substances that nevertheless exert a curative or ameliorating effect via the powerful means of suggestion. Down the ages, the placebo effect has been the doctors' most formidable ally. (Oddly enough, even when patients are told that what they are receiving is a mere placebo, with no true curative action of its own, they experience more relief than if they are given nothing.)

There is another reason, apart from the ethical prohibition, why doctors no longer prescribe inert placebos for their patients: the faint hope that a real drug will actually do some good. After all, diagnosis is not an exact science, and in the majority of patients who have nothing much wrong with them and who present themselves to a doctor, the absence of illness is not proved beyond reasonable doubt. Therefore, a drug that would do them good if they had the disease they are most likely to have, if they had a disease at all, seems the best bet in the circumstances.

Thus too free an access to doctors is likely to result in the excessive consumption of medicaments, with all the attendant side effects. Psychological discomfort is thus often transformed into physical discomfort. But access to doctors that is too difficult also has its drawbacks, which are too obvious to need enumeration.

In Britain, with considerable ingenuity, we seem to have to have achieved the worst of both worlds: for it is both too easy and too difficult to see a doctor. This seems paradoxical, but in reality is not. For some it is too difficult to see a doctor because for others it is too easy.

The apparent paradox needs an explanation. Every British doctor is aware that a very high percentage of his patients have little objective medical need to see him. They attend his office for the same reason that Mallory tried to climb Everest: because it is there. They go to the doctor because they have no reason not to go to the doctor. There is no fee to deter them, or make them think whether their visit is really necessary, and no social disapprobation either for wasting the doctor's time. Indeed, in the current non-judgemental climate of opinion, a man's desire to go to the doctor is *ipso facto* proof that he has a good reason to do so. The time a doctor can devote to his patients being inelastic, his time spent on trifling matters naturally reduces the time he can devote to serious ones.

That people are perfectly well able to distinguish the serious from the trivial was impressed upon me recently during a visit to Belgrade, in the aftermath of NATO's bombing campaign. I visited the ambulance service there and met its director. He told me that when the ambulance service in Serbia received an emergency call from a patient, a doctor was dispatched in the ambulance to attend him. During the bombing campaign, there was a most curious decline in the use of the service, by about 50 per cent. Moreover, the percentage of calls estimated by the doctors dispatched on the ambulances to have been medically necessary doubled, from about half to nearly 100 per cent. This more or less proves that people (at least in Serbia) are perfectly well aware of the difference in the significance of a heart attack and a panic attack, if circumstances force them to think about it. And there is no reason to suppose that the Serbs differ in this capacity from the rest of humanity.

(There were other most interesting facts to be gleaned from the records of the Serbian ambulance service. During the bombing, the number of injuries in Belgrade declined precipitously, which is precisely the opposite of what one might have expected. In part, no doubt, this was because activities that often result in injuries – such as driving, factory work and so forth – declined. But it also probably indicates that one of the most important causes of injury in modern life – that is to say, self-infliction – also declined. Thus war, sad to relate, appears to be an answer – or more exactly, one answer among other possible answers – to Man's existential problems. In the absence of war, the self-infliction of injury and illness is another.)

It seems, then, that too ready an access to doctors is – in ordinary circumstances, and given the nature of human nature – something not to be wished. It is an open invitation to waste doctors' time, and has potentially serious consequences for those who are seriously ill. Not only will it delay the treatment of the latter, but doctors will become so accustomed to the fact that there is nothing seriously wrong with the majority of their patients that they will be more likely to dismiss the complaints of those who actually have something wrong with them.

But how is access to doctors to be limited, in such a way that the sick are not deterred from visiting them, but the bored, fractious and self-obsessed are? If the means of deterrence used is payment, and there seem to be few alternatives, the spectre of impoverished old people dying for want of medical care is raised. Better that a doctor should be consulted a thousand times unnecessarily than that one old person should fail to attend because of inability to pay. And here we come to the thorny question of equity and justice in the provision of health-care, which so obsesses us.

The first step is to dismiss out of hand the absurd idea that anyone has a right to healthcare. No one has a right to health-care. Indeed, where could such a right come from? The increasing tendency in modern society to treat all goods, and all human desiderata, as the American Declaration of Independence treats life, liberty and the pursuit of happiness is extremely foolish, for reasons I shall explain. The problem of the metaphysical origin of human rights will not go away. It should be remembered that the American Declaration of Independence asserted the rights to life, liberty and the pursuit of happiness in the belief that all men were created equal and that these rights were endowed upon them by their creator. In other words, the Declaration was, if not a religious, then at least a theist, document. Take away God, and the origin of the rights asserted becomes completely mysterious.

If we do not believe in God (and of course it is also perfectly possible to believe in God without believing in the right to life, liberty and the pursuit of human happiness, or in any other rights whatsoever), we have to find some other transcendent source of our supposed human rights. And the fact is that, while an ever-increasing proportion of the population believes it has rights, of ever-growing number and complexity into the bargain, an ever-decreasing proportion of the population believes in God.

It might, of course, be argued that the source of our rights is in our human nature. But there are undoubted difficulties in this view of the matter. The headhunters of Borneo are indubitably human, but they do not believe in (and would not even understand) the right to freedom of religious worship, let alone the right to healthcare. What we believe to be our rights are in fact the philosophical product of a particular culture at a particular time. But rights must, by the very nature of the concept, transcend both culture and time: they are universal, or they are nothing. Either we must believe that our society has discovered pre-existing rights, rather as Koch discovered the tubercle bacillus, and that therefore we stand at the pinnacle of the history of human moral endeavour, or that in fact our supposed rights are fictions, which we made up to suit ourselves. In the former case we are guilty of the most terrible arrogance (though, interestingly, those who most strongly believe in human rights also pay most lip-service to the contradictory ideal of multiculturalism), while in the latter case we are reduced to lying and pretence. We pretend the rights we have awarded ourselves (or that governments have awarded us) have transcendent origins, but we know perfectly well that they have not. Like most pretences, this one can be kept up a while, so long as no one agrees to talk about the metaphysical legerdemain, but not for ever. The truth will out, with a consequent loss of faith and an access of moral confusion.

If there is a right to tangible goods (such as food, housing and healthcare), someone has an obligation to provide them, since they do not arrive as free gifts of God or nature. They are, in fact, the products of human labour. The obligation to provide others with the fruit of one's labour is indistinguishable from slavery – except that one has the option to do nothing, since food, housing and healthcare (among other necessities and desiderata) are one's rights. A man who chooses not to work therefore merely shifts the responsibility for providing these things from himself to others, as it must be his right to do if these things are in themselves truly rights.

The idea that tangible benefits are and should be conferred as of right exerts a most lamentable effect upon the human personality. The reason for this is obvious. In a world of rights, there is no reason for gratitude or indeed for kindness. Social arrangements will be so perfect than no one will need to be good: nor, of course, can there be any dire consequences for those who are bad. There is no reason to be grateful for what is received as of right, since it is precisely that – a right. At the same time, resentment is aroused when those things which are believed to be rights (an ever-increasing number) are not received. Neither ingratitude nor resentment is an attractive human characteristic: and the consequences of the doctrine of rights, with its attendant ingratitude and resentment, are to be seen in British hospitals. A right being by its nature inalienable, it does not matter how its possessor behaves: he can smash up a house and demand a new one ('It's my right'), and he can abuse and assault hospital staff and demand medical attention ('It's my right'). In these circumstances, therefore, it is not surprising that 40 per cent of British general practitioners are assaulted by at least one patient a year, or that a nursing sister to whom I spoke recently told me that a patient in her ward informed her, after she had been assaulted by another of her patients, that this was what she was paid for.

There is, and can be, no general right to healthcare.

It does not follow in the least, of course, that healthcare should not be available for people. The satisfaction of rights does not exhaust moral duties. A society in which the ill are well treated is better (at least in this regard, though not necessarily in others, since health is not the whole purpose of human existence) than one in which they are not. No one would want to see a society in which the ill were denied help: but this is because human kindness, decency, solidarity and sympathy demand that we succour the sick, not because the sick have rights.

The question of how healthcare should be provided cannot be answered by an appeal to a single simple desideratum: for example, that everyone should receive the same level of healthcare, in the name of equality or equity. Equality is not much of a value in itself, for it would be satisfied by a system in which everyone received the same appalling healthcare and died at the same early age. Would a society in which no one received good healthcare be better than one in which half the population did? Egalitarians, but surely no sensible person, would answer that it would.

At the very least, egalitarians would have to add a condition to their demand for equality: that the healthcare to which all should have equal access must be good, or better than good. But in that case, equality is no longer the sole moral yardstick by which a healthcare system should be measured. If an unequal system nevertheless provided a better overall level of care, then it might with reason be preferred to one that gave the same, but inferior, level of care to everyone.

It would nevertheless be true to say that our medical journals and departments of social medicine exhibit an obsession with equality as a value. Week after week, for example, both the *Lancet* and the *British Medical Journal* expatiate the evils of inequality, usually with the implication that there should be more central planning and taxation to even out the inequalities (which they invariably consider inequities also). It isn't difficult to demonstrate that, in the last analysis, the only regime of which the editorialists of these august scientific periodicals – with a combined circulation of about a million – approve is that of Cuba under Fidel.

Equality is equated by these journals with justice. Any inequality is therefore *ipso facto* a sign of injustice; and the greater the inequality, the greater the injustice. No attempt is ever made to distinguish between injustice and unfairness: they are conflated, the better to arouse the emotions of the reader. The journals are nothing if not consistent: they not only decry any inequality within society, but decry inequalities between societies. What they propose as a solution on a national level they do no hesitate to propose on a global one. The editors of medical journals and heads of university departments of social medicine are the would-be philosopher-kings of our time.

In several years, I have seen no examination of equality as a desideratum in any medical publication: its complete beneficence is assumed, as if no sensible, or at least decent, person could fail to approve of it. This is despite the fact that a very few obvious considerations cast doubt upon the identity of justice and equality. I am not a philosopher by training, but it is not difficult to see objections to equality as a desirable outcome.

By definition, justice must take deserts into account: otherwise the Red Queen's demand that the sentence should come before the verdict would make perfect sense. But it is clear that not everyone's deserts are equal: the diligent and the lazy, the honest and the dishonest, the violent and the peaceful, the clever and the stupid, the selfless and the selfish. If everyone were to receive the same reward for very different conduct, the meaning of life – or such meaning as we are able to give it – would be destroyed utterly. Indeed, there could be no greater injustice than equality of outcome.

There is, of course, a sense in which a doctor must believe in equality, though not for its own sake: he must treat all his patients to the best of his ability, without distinguishing between them on moral grounds. It cannot be that he likes all of them equally, or invariably approves of their way of life. Some may be out-and-out criminals: the thought that the world would be a better place without one or other of his patients must never occur to him, or if it does (the mind not being able to live up to its own high ethical standards), he must not act upon it. The fact that doctors, being fallible and human, are likely to make more strenuous efforts on behalf of those with whom they feel sympathy than on behalf of those towards whom they feel antipathy should not obscure the fact that, ideally, doctors make no distinctions between their patients. Again, it is true that medical considerations sometimes merge imperceptibly into moral ones, as when, for example, cardiac surgeons refuse to perform coronary bypass operations upon people who refuse to give up smoking: for it is difficult entirely to believe that the surgeons involved are passing no derogatory moral judgement upon the patients upon whom they do not operate (nor is their judgement necessarily wrong in itself). But on the whole it is not the doctor's place to tailor his treatment to his patient's moral worth. A VD clinic is not the place for sexual censoriousness.

But the kind of equality that the doctor must practise has nothing to do with the kind of equality demanded by the medical journals. If he does not try to do his best for his patients, the doctor fails in his most elementary duty, which is to help people. Indeed, he could hardly be a doctor unless he took this stance. It may be that doing his best for patients requires the doctor to act differently according to the needs, desires and capacities of his individual patients, but that is another matter. All his patients are equal in the sense that he does his best for them.

The equality of the journals of departments of social medicine is very different from the doctor's clinical egalitarianism.

It is not adventitious, as the practising doctor's is: it does not depend upon who happens to present himself at his own behest to the doctor for treatment. Rather, it is the demand that everyone should die at the same age or suffer the same illnesses. It not an ethical equality that is demanded, but a statistical one.

Recently a publisher sent me a small book by a professor of public health,the cover of which bore the startling words 'Inequality kills'. The book was pretty much a conspectus of what is now the orthodox medical view of equality. My own view of the author's underlying intentions – though of course I cannot prove it beyond reasonable doubt – is that he was making an intellectualised plea for increased funding and power for people like himself, to exercise more and more control over everyone else's lives: for their own good, of course. Indeed, it would hardly be going too far to say that the book was a plea for medical totalitarianism.

The populations of those countries with small differentials in personal income, said the author, have longer life expectancies than the populations of those countries at approximately the same level of economic development with large differentials in personal income. For example, Swedes and Canadians live longer than Americans. Ergo, inequality kills.

The author acknowledges that a statistical correlation does not necessarily imply a causative relationship. He therefore proposes a mechanism by which inequality kills. He does not believe that physical or financial deprivation is the explanation, because even the poorest in the United States have access to comforts and goods that would have made Croesus envious. Rather, it is relative poverty that kills – a poor person being someone with an income of less than half the average for his society. (This rather strange and arbitrary definition, of course, means that a society composed solely of millionaires, or even of billionaires, would not necessarily be free of poverty, if the income distribution were nevertheless sufficiently unequal. But let it pass.)

How, then, does relative poverty of the kind seen in the United States and other unequal societies kill? The answer proposed is via the stress caused by the comparison of oneself with people higher up the social or economic scale. This induces a depressed or despondent state of mind, which in turn affects the endocrine system, particularly the excretion of corticosteroids. When these are chronically raised because of the continual psychological distress caused by what amounts to envy (but of course is never actually called this by the author), the immune system is adversely affected. The stressed person is susceptible to infections that would otherwise be resisted and overcome: hence the increased rate of infectious disease among the relatively poor, even in times when infectious disease is no longer the leading cause of death. The fact that the relatively poor also have higher rates of diabetes, high blood pressure, coronary artery disease and stroke is likewise accounted for, because high levels of circulating corticosteroids have these effects. (The author rather forgets that, not so very many years ago, an increased rate of heart attacks in a population was regarded as a sign of prosperity, not of poverty; and indeed, in some populations, such as the Gujarati, heart attacks occur principally among the prosperous, not among the poor.)

Egalitarian societies do not stress their populations psychologically as unequal ones do: hence their lower death rates and higher life expectancies. The correlation between an equal income distribution and a higher life expectancy is thus a causative one. The solution (for those countries with high death rates and low life expectancies) is twofold: first, unequal societies should become equal, by means of increased taxation, and second, an egalitarian system of socialised medicine should be generously funded.

On this view, of course, a decreased death rate and an increased life expectancy are so desirable in themselves that all social and economic arrangements should be directed towards procuring them, no matter at what other cost, including the suppression of freedom.

What is omitted from the paean of praise of egalitarianism is the fact that the differences between, say, Sweden and the United States are not in fact very large. The life expectancy in Sweden is perhaps two years longer than in the United States: two years out of seventy-nine. Nor are the two societies in other ways comparable: the city of New York alone has twice the population of Sweden, and is full of immigrants, many of whom have arrived from conditions that may have damaged them for life. The massive upheavals that would be required to turn the United States into a larger Sweden would at best result in a relatively trivial gain, and might easily have quite the opposite effect.

The country with the highest life expectancy of all, Japan, is surely not plausibly described as egalitarian, even if (as is far from certain) its income differentials are comparatively small. On the contrary, it is the country *par excellence* of hierarchy, in which an inferior cannot contradict a superior under any circumstances. It is, after all, a very crude view of human social relations to suppose that equality of income must necessarily produce equality in social relations. What perhaps is different about Japan is the acceptance of hierarchy, as being natural, inescapable and necessary for the welfare of society.

If this were the case, then equalising income would not be the only way of improving the health of an unequal population. It would make as much sense, or more, to preach the necessity of inequality, so that people accepted it with a good grace, instead of being eaten up by envy and resentment, as they are at present. Indeed, if it is envy and resentment which kill, rather than inequality per se, those who preach egalitarianism and the moral illegitimacy of inequality and hierarchy are responsible for death and disease.

Not, of course, that the acceptance of hierarchy and inequality, let alone the things themselves, can be defended on the grounds that they are conducive to health.

The most egalitarian system of healthcare is generally regarded as the system prevailing in Cuba or in Britain, which is provided out of central government funds and is free to the patient at the point of use. The Cuban system is more egalitarian than the British, of course, because Britain retains a private sector, which is used by 5 or 10 per cent of the population, and there are moreover charges for prescriptions (except for the old, for children, for the chronic sick and for the unemployed: that is to say, 90 per cent of the people who need prescriptions in the first place). The special clinics for leaders in Cuba, by contrast, are used by a mere handful, nothing like 5 or 10 per cent of the population.

The British National Health System has been in operation since 1948, but has not so far done anything to reduce the inequalities in health between the richest and poorest sections of the population. Indeed, it is commonly accepted wisdom that the inequalities have increased in latter years rather than grown smaller. A relative deterioration is often presented as if it were an absolute one, usually for polemical reasons. At any rate, the usual response to the increasing gap between the health of the rich and the poor is to propose more spending on the very system that has failed to reduce the gap in half a century. It is as if the intrinsic merit of the system had been imprinted at birth on the brains of the British, as goslings have imprinted upon their brains the image of the first thing they see after their birth, which they follow blindly, irrespective of the totally inappropriate nature of their filial devotions. You can still sometimes hear it said that the NHS is the envy of the world, though I have travelled to eighty countries and have never encountered any envy of it. It has even been called the only institution to which Britons now feel any loyalty.

The NHS was predicated on the supposition that healthcare was not a good as other goods are, to be rationed by price. Healthcare was in a different moral category from, say, food or automobiles. Unlike all other goods, it was the *sine qua non* of the good life, and therefore was to be removed from the marketplace, which was so capricious and unequal in the granting of its favours. Henceforth, everyone was to receive exactly the care he needed, regardless of his ability to pay. There is no denying the simple nobility of the aim, however it turned out in practice.

But as we have seen, an egalitarian institution did not render egalitarian results. Although the health of everyone improved (as it did everywhere else in the developed world), the health advantages of wealth did not disappear, but seemed rather to increase. Why?

In the first place, as I have already mentioned, the health-care system determines the health of a population, and presumably of subgroups of that population, only to a limited extent. In the second place, the equality of care provided to the middle and lower classes under the NHS is more notional and theoretical than real and practical. This itself is for a number of reasons, among them the fact that the middle classes know better how to take advantage of what the system offers. Doctors, the most important group of employees in the system, are themselves members of the middle classes, not merely by virtue of their occupation, but usually by birth as well. Many middle-class people therefore have relatives or friends who are doctors, and human nature being imperfect, it is only to be expected that favours are asked for and conferred. If there is a queue caused by shortages within the system, middle-class people know how to jump it.

Moreover, they can assure themselves of the best of whatever is going by being vociferous, argumentative, querulous and even litigious. Such people are better able to get what they want than people who can barely string a sentence together or write a coherent letter of complaint. Everyone who works in public services wants a quiet life, and the easiest way to achieve it is by satisfying the most vocal members of the public. They used to say in Africa that the death of one white man will cause more trouble than the death of a thousand Africans; likewise, in the NHS, the unjustified complaint of one bourgeois will cause more trouble than the justified though ill-expressed, badly written and orthographically unsound complaints of a hundred members of the lower classes. Insofar as the NHS has benefited anyone, it has benefited the middle classes, who were already well catered for before the NHS was instituted.

Is the NHS a success or not? There is not a simple answer to this question. Judged by the standards of health that prevail in roughly comparable countries, Britain is neither marvellous nor terrible, but about average. It is often now reported in the press that Britain lags severely behind its competitors in the treatment of cancer and cardiovascular disease, but there are grounds for scepticism. After all, cancer and cardiovascular disease account between them for three-quarters of all deaths in developed countries, and if Britain were very much worse in the treatment of them than other such countries, one might expect this deficiency to be reflected in poor comparative figures for life expectancy. In fact, in this respect Britain is slightly better than Germany and Denmark, two countries held up as being advanced in their treatment of cancer and cardiovascular disease. The differences must be relatively small, therefore.

It is often stated that the NHS is cheap, at least by international standards, though in absolute terms the sums expended on it seem vast indeed. And since the health indices of Britain are approximately those of countries that spend a far higher percentage of their gross national products on healthcare, it is deemed to be extremely efficient. In healthcare expenditure there appears to be a law of diminishing returns: it becomes ever costlier to produce a tangible health benefit. Nothing is easier than to waste money on healthcare.

In actual fact, the British state spends about the same proportion of GNP on healthcare as other comparable states: but because of the ideology of the NHS, that it is a free and comprehensive service that is supposed to meet all the health needs of the population, there has been a reluctance on the part of the population to spend its own income after tax on private healthcare. The difference in healthcare expenditure between Britain and other developed countries is therefore not in the state but in the private sector.

The acceptance of the ideology has been virtually universal. I remember a retired man of comfortable means who had waited several years for his hernia operation on the NHS (by no means an uncommon experience). The hernia caused him considerable discomfort, so I asked him why, since he was well able to afford it, he did not have it operated upon privately. His discomfort would then be over in a matter of weeks. He replied that he had paid his taxes for many years, often at a high, indeed confiscatory, rate, and that he was damned if he was going to let the state off its obligations to him. Why should he have paid all those taxes to receive nothing in return? He had been told that one of the benefits of the high rate was a free and comprehensive healthcare system: well, he was going to take advantage of it, even if it killed him.

There is one great advantage of the healthcare system paid for entirely, or almost entirely, by the state: the doctors are salaried, and therefore have no pecuniary interest in over-investigating or in over-treating their patients. Of course, for this to be so, the doctors' salaries must be at a sufficiently high level that the doctors are able to live satisfactorily on them, for otherwise the system would descend into communist-type corruption, in which lowly paid doctors eke out their incomes by taking bribes from patients. Under the Soviet system, what appeared to be a free and universal healthcare system was in practice no such thing: doctors had to be paid (usually in kind, for the economy was in large part demonetarised) for appointments, examinations and treatment; and nurses likewise had to be paid to deliver the treatment ordered by the doctor. One reads in the medical press laments over the worsening health conditions in Russia (where the life expectancy of men in particular has undergone a spectacular and unprecedented decline), as if the worsening had been caused by the destruction of the free, universal and comprehensive healthcare system – which is also often claimed as one of the few achievements of the revolution. But that service was never as described by idealists. No doubt health services have deteriorated greatly in Russia and other states of the former Soviet Union (I have seen this for myself), but for reasons that have more to do with the unreformability of the Gogolian-Leninist state than with the abandonment of free medical care that was never free.

In the British system, by contrast, there has been very little corruption, at least by the standards prevailing in the rest of human history. Most doctors and nurses in the NHS perform their duties conscientiously and to the best of their ability. It is true that there have been reports of senior doctors deliberately keeping their waiting lists on the NHS long to promote their private practices, and thus their incomes, but – though I have worked in the system on and off for over a quarter of a century – I have known very few cases of such behaviour, which is easier to allege than to prove. The one speciality in which such behaviour seems prevalent is dermatology, for it is a fact that almost everyone is prepared, despite the ideology of the NHS, to pay for the preservation of his appearance. Even quite poor people, who would never consider paying to see any other kind of specialist, are prepared to make the sacrifice on behalf of their skin: an unblemished appearance being more important to Man than life itself. Three factors contribute to the exceptionalism of dermatology within the British system: first is the importance people place on the physical presentation of themselves to others; second is the relatively limited sums that can be spent on dermatology, which uses few expensive procedures, unlike, say, cardiology; and third is the very inadequate number of dermatologists in Britain. There are five thousand senior dermatologists in Germany, but only three hundred in Britain. That they have long waiting lists is therefore hardly surprising, and not necessarily a sign of villainy on their part. In Germany, you can get a dermatological opinion in a day; in Britain, you are lucky if you can get one, even privately, in under a month. It is simply a matter of demand and supply, the latter being totally insufficient in Britain. As for the reason for this insufficiency of dermatologists, it has probably something to do with the puritanical nature of the bureaucrats who control the state system. Few are the diseases of the skin with a fatal outcome, or that even cause physical pain and discomfort. In a certain restricted sense, therefore, they are trivial: they will never show up in the figures for death rates or life expectancy. On the basis, therefore, that scarce resources must be carefully husbanded, dermatology can safely be neglected. Sufferers from disfiguring skin conditions are unlikely to form a strong pressure group precisely because of their disfigurement, and so the shortage will never obtrude much upon public consciousness. Each sufferer from a skin condition, who is unable to see a dermatologist for several months, suffers alone.

There is little doubt that the NHS, while it treats most diseases as they should be treated, and prevents most deaths that should be prevented, does so in conditions that are pretty wretched for a society that calls itself wealthy. It is a system better adapted to a poor society, in which people have no disposable income, are unaccustomed by their housing conditions to privacy, and so forth, than to a society in which many millions go abroad on holidays, the majority own their homes, have more than one car per family, have a video in every room, and so forth. The fact is that everyone who enters a National Health Service hospital is *ipso facto* a pauper. He might be a well or badly treated pauper, but a pauper he is. He may indeed be a millionaire, but he must still accept what he is given. He has no choice (other than to reject treatment altogether).

About thirty years ago, at the outset of my career, while I was still a student, the father of a friend of mine, who was a local general practitioner, was brought to the casualty department of the hospital in which I was working. He had a very serious condition, from which he subsequently died. Unfortunately, there were no beds immediately available in the hospital, and so he was obliged to wait in the corridor on a bed trolley for several hours until one became available. I remember thinking how humiliating this must have been for him (or for anyone else, for that matter). The fact that he was a medical colleague availed him nothing: the hospital was simply too full for any special privileges to be granted him on account of his membership of the medical profession.

No doubt there are some who would see inspiration in this story. The doctor's relatively privileged social position did not spare him the humiliations inflicted upon the rest of the population by a system of constant shortage: and this is justice of a kind. It is a strange fact that the British see in the discomforts and humiliations of their system of medical care a guarantee that it is just and fair. They don't seem to care much if they suffer, so long as the next man suffers as much as they do.

The problems of the NHS are not new. From the very moment of its inception, the NHS was storing up problems for the near future. Its supporters paint a picture of the pre-NHS era in Britain as though it were some terrible dark age, in which no one – apart from the rich – was ever treated. This is not so: by the time of the First World War, three-quarters of the population were medically insured, and voluntary hospitals provided attention for the indigent. (It is, however, true that much medical treatment until the second half of the twentieth century must have been of doubtful benefit, beyond the placebo effect.) The fact is that the institution of the NHS brought investment in new hospitals in Britain to an almost immediate stop: which is why, even today, there is scarcely a hospital in the country that is not a patchwork of miscellaneous buildings, with little jerry-built accretions added on as miserly funds became available in dribs and drabs. The overall impression given by British hospitals is one of poverty, of a country struggling against fearful odds to provide at least minimal medical care for its impoverished population. So continual and unremitting has the financial crisis of the NHS been that it has never given consideration to any but the most utilitarian purposes, so that all British hospitals, even the newest, are aesthetic nightmares. No new hospitals in Britain equal in appearance those of Turkey, let alone those of the United States.

Thirty years after my friend's father was left on a trolley in the corridor of the hospital in which I was working, I find that I would be in precisely the same situation as my friend's father, if I were to suffer like him from a medical emergency. Like him, I would have to go to my local hospital, where the wait for a bed to become available has, if anything, lengthened in the meantime. It is not uncommon at busy periods for patients to spend an entire day on a hospital trolley, at least if it is adjudged that they will not die during that period. There is no way by which, under the NHS, I can avoid this humiliation: I cannot say I want to go to another hospital, but even if I could, there would be little point in doing so since they are all in precisely the same position. I might as well wait in one corridor as another. I cannot pay to insure myself against the humiliations that would be visited upon me by the NHS (not deliberately or sadistically, I hasten to add) because the local private hospitals are not equipped to deal with medical emergencies. On the contrary, they treat mainly the chronic conditions that the NHS takes so long to treat.

Once a bed is found for me, I must be grateful for it. In my hospital, it would most likely be in a Nightingale ward, that is to say, in a ward in which two rows of beds are lined up against the wall of a very long chamber. It cannot be said that anyone dies because of being in such a ward, and perhaps such wards even have advantages, at least at times when there are shortages of nurses: for a single nurse can take in at a glance what is happening to a lot of patients.

Nevertheless, the prospect of admission to such a ward thoroughly daunts me. There is a complete lack of privacy that curtains drawn round the bed cannot correct. (There are two ways of announcing death in a Nightingale ward: the first is to draw the curtains round the recently deceased's bed; the second is to draw the curtains round everyone else's bed.) In the last few years it has been decided to integrate British wards sexually: one end or side for males, the other for females. Needless to say, this integration was instituted by hospital managers without reference to the patients themselves, who almost certainly did not want it. The fact that their wishes in the matter were neither adhered to nor even properly ascertained is highly symbolic of the relationship of patients to the NHS: as of paupers to the parish fathers.

The din in Nightingale wards is, of course, nearly continual. The television is on for eighteen hours a day, and it is quite impossible to extinguish it, even if no one in the ward actually wants to watch it. You can try turning it off, as I have on several occasions, but within three minutes at the most someone – though it is always impossible to discover who – will have turned it back on again. Imagine waking up from an operation to find a drivelling chat show being poured into your ear; or being paralysed down one side of your body after a stroke, to be subjected compulsorily to a televised keep-fit class conducted to pop music by an Amazonian taskmistress in a Lycra leotard.

Worse still, the television is seldom unopposed by other electronic forms of entertainment, equally compulsory for the unfortunate patient. The nurses these days often have music playing from tape recorders at their work stations: they claim not to be able to concentrate without it. Needless to say, the music they play is not of the type that has charms to soothe the savage breast: on the contrary, it is usually of the kind to arouse the breast to savagery.

Patients shriek or snore; through no fault of their own, they often emit the most undignified sounds, to say nothing of other emissions. To all of this, the NHS patient is necessarily subjected.

If he wants to make a telephone call, the patient cannot do so in privacy, but rather for the whole ward to hear. The public telephone is paraded around the ward like the cart that bears a statue of a Hindu god.

The patient is harried from his bed the moment he will no longer die if he is discharged. No question of kindness to him is allowed to delay his departure, or get in the way of as swift a turnover of patients as possible. The policy is definitely to discharge patients quicker but sicker, as they say in America. If it turns out that the patient is discharged prematurely, and has to be readmitted because of complications that have arisen from his premature discharge, so much the better, at least for the hospital statistics. It can be claimed that two episodes of illness have been treated instead of one, neither of them having required a prolonged stay in hospital.

Of course, since most of us spend very little time in hospital, the deficiencies I have outlined above do not loom very large in our lives. Nevertheless, they make being ill an even more unpleasant experience than it need be, and there is absolutely no prospect that the deficiencies will ever be eliminated under the NHS as it is at present constituted. The kind of expenditure necessary to provide services more appropriate to a wealthy and sophisticated society is a political and economic impossibility. The British must accept their pauperisation, or find another way of funding their healthcare.

Moreover, the state as monopoly provider of healthcare has the authority and the power to dictate to both the doctor and the patient what treatment the patient should have. For a long time, the state in Britain did not exercise this power, but was content to let the medical profession remain in control, as an independent, liberal, learned profession. But as medical treatment has grown ever more expensive, and as governments have shown ever less inclination to allow any part of society to regulate itself, so doctors are being forced more and more to do what governments dictate, and less and less what they, as individual members of the profession, think they ought to do. After all, the government, as keeper of the public purse that pays doctors, has the duty to ensure that the public is getting value for money. How else can it ensure this other than by telling doctors what to do?

Not surprisingly, the result has been an increasing and quite swift demoralisation of the medical profession. Traditionally, it has been difficult to get into medical school: only the academically gifted, or at least the academically determined, have been able to do so. The medical course is demanding and arduous; postgraduate training is often even worse, requiring not only long hours of study, but many disturbed nights spent on duty. There is probably no profession more arduously trained. And the reward at the end of all this? Increasingly, doctors are treated as lowly technicians, whose job is simply to implement instructions sent to them by government committees. They are not in a position to refuse. It is small wonder that, in Britain, three-quarters of all senior doctors want to retire as soon as possible, and a half of newly graduated doctors wish they had never taken up medicine as a career. Intelligent people want to be independent, not clerks and bureaucrats. This does not bode well for the future of medical care in Britain. Already fewer young people are applying to medical schools, and soon they will be of lower intellectual calibre than formerly. The time will come when only very second-rate care will be available for the majority in Britain, while the élite, as in much of Africa and the Third World, will travel elsewhere for better medical treatment.

In summary, then, a state-funded system such as the British NHS is for the moment capable of providing at least a bare minimum of healthcare to its population. That population is given no choice in the matter of its treatment, other than that of rejecting it altogether, and is pauperised by the system, even when the people who work in it are dedicated (as most of them are) to the welfare of their patients. Its overall cost in comparative terms is not high. But the governmental source of funding is fast eroding the independence of the medical profession, a process that will eventually have serious consequences for the quality of medical care. Funding from general taxation has also meant that almost all services are delivered as cheaply as possible, in depressing and even degrading surroundings.

Furthermore, technical medical progress (which almost always leads to an increase in cost, at least initially) invariably represents a crisis for a system such as the NHS, because of the inflexibility of the system's funding. The money necessary to pay for new methods of treatment, when forthcoming at all, must be withdrawn from some other part of the budget: Peter must always be robbed to pay Paul. Thus the accurate impression is given that the NHS is always limping reluctantly after progress. It would be better for the NHS if no new treatments were ever discovered.

What, though, of systems of healthcare with a privately funded component (there is nowhere in the world where a purely private system reigns)? Have they no disadvantages?

First, of course, is the fear that, where money changes hands, doctors will act in their own interests rather than in those of their patients. They needn't be scoundrels for this to happen: the human mind is quite subtle enough to be able to persuade itself that something that it would like to do is actually in the interests of someone else, without any overtly fraudulent plan being consciously formed. It has been repeatedly found that, in different areas of the United States, the frequency of certain operations (hysterectomy, for example) is more directly proportional to the number of surgeons performing them than to the incidence of pathology necessitating them. The surgeons, with one or two exceptions, no doubt, are not charlatans or shysters: in each individual case, they have assuredly persuaded themselves of the clinical rightness of what they were about to do.

At the same time, such willingness to treat quickly and aggressively can also work in the patient's favour, where such treatment actually produces a clear benefit.

There are, of course, ethical objections to systems of healthcare in which payment by the patient is involved. People differ in their ability to pay; some are not able to pay at all. Why should the best – or at least, the most expensive – treatment go only, or principally, to the rich?

This objection depends upon health and healthcare being goods of a different class from all other goods. It is also incipiently totalitarian. After all, healthcare services are not the major determinant of the health of any population. If it can be shown, for example, that what people eat and the houses they live in affect their health either positively or negatively, it would, according to the doctrine of health as a good distinct from all others, be incumbent upon the government to provide the food and housing conditions that resulted in the best health. Certain cars survive accidents better than others: should, therefore, the safer (and usually larger and more expensive) cars be provided for everyone who wishes to drive at all? A brief glance through any general medical journal, or any journal of epidemiology, will demonstrate that there are an infinite number of factors that affect health, some of them more deeply than any likely differences in medical treatment that people receive. If private expenditure on healthcare should be forbidden on the grounds that health is too fundamentally important from the ethical point of view to be left to market forces, then almost everything else – for example, the food supply – should be excluded from the play of market forces also. This explains why the market is never referred to in the medical journals except as a term of abuse and scorn, and why references to Cuba are almost always favourable. There is no market in Cuba, and until recently its health services were held up as models of what central planning and implementation could achieve when freed of the exigencies of the marketplace. What is omitted from the paeans of praise is the fact that Cuba, at the time of its revolution, was already the second-healthiest place in Latin America (after Argentina), with a well-developed, if uneven, infrastructure of healthcare. It is also conveniently forgotten that the healthcare system in Cuba was dependent upon massive subsidy from the Soviet Union, without which it could not have operated. Not everywhere in the world can be subsidised in this fashion, unless generous benefactors on Mars be found.

But private healthcare suffers from some of the same pressures as state-funded healthcare. This is because private healthcare, like state healthcare, is generally funded through a third party, not by direct payment of the doctor by the patient. In the case of private healthcare, the third party is an insurance company, which in the United States has begun to act in much the same way as the state in Britain. The insurance company wants increasingly to control what doctors do, both to contain its costs and to increase its profit margins. The doctors in the United States are therefore suffering from the same kind of demoralisation as they are suffering in Britain. Insofar as there are many different insurance companies, each operating different schemes of coverage, the situation is less serious for them: because a monolith weighs more heavily than several megaliths. But the reason for their present discontent has fundamental similarities. As in Britain, fewer young people are applying for admission to medical schools.

Insurance schemes are necessary because modern sophisticated healthcare is so expensive that few individuals could pay for it out of their disposable assets, when the need for it arises. Only the very rich can afford to pay hospital bills for complex surgical procedures directly from their pockets.

Of course, insurance works on the principle that what is insured against is unlikely to happen to any given individual. Health insurance covers the cost – the very large cost – of a liver transplant only because liver transplants are rarely necessary. If they were too frequently necessary, the cost of insurance premiums would itself be prohibitive. The result is that most people's insurance goes to pay for someone else's care (as well as, of course, for a margin of profit for the insurance company). A man who dies in his bed suddenly after a long life in which he has not suffered a day's serious illness but who has paid large insurance contributions will have wasted a large proportion of his income.

To avoid this wastage, and to restore the direct nature of the patient-doctor consultation without the intrusion of third parties into it, a scheme has been devised in the United States in which a person puts a certain part of his income in a special savings account, whose deposits are to be used solely for medical purposes. By the time he needs expensive medical treatment (and 90 per cent of medical expenses are incurred in old age), it is hoped that the patient will have accumulated enough in his savings account to pay for treatment directly. The patient will choose his doctor, and his doctor will advise him as he believes best, not as the government or insurance company directs him to advise.

Of course, under such a scheme there will need to be a component of insurance, especially in the first years of a person's health savings account, because it is possible – though statistically unlikely – that he will fall ill before he has accumulated very much, and because it is always possible that the cost of necessary treatment will exceed the total amount saved. But at the end of a person's life, if he has not spent all his health savings on medical care, he will be able to leave the remainder to his heirs.

Some people would never be able to save very much, because they were permanently unemployed or because they never earned very much in the first place. Obviously, some kind of public provision would have to be made for the incapable, at least in a civilised society. But it is worth recalling that we in Britain are already paying something like 12 per cent of our annual incomes to the government so that it might provide healthcare for us, as it sees fit. Paid into private funds, controlled by individuals, there would be some hope of genuine competition enforcing efficiency and value for money on the providers of healthcare. Under a system of government monopoly, by contrast, all attempts to increase efficiency decrease it, and all attempts to cut bureaucracy add to it. The same is likely to be true, though perhaps to a lesser extent, of insurance companies. A bureaucracy does not cease to be a bureaucracy merely because it is also a private company.

A doctor who works as an individual contractor to the

patient, rather than as a salaried member of a bureaucratic machine, is likely in the long run to be more satisfied with his work, even at precisely the same level of income. Independence is one of the most important determinants of job satisfaction. I know from personal experience that being paid extra for getting out of bed at night to attend a patient is slightly less unpleasant than not being paid extra for getting out of bed at night to attend a patient (I have experienced both). And when a doctor is dependent upon a good reputation among his patients for future work, he is likely to be better mannered than when he knows his patients have to come to him because he is their government-allocated doctor. The patients' lack of choice gives him a power over them that he might choose not to abuse because he has the requisite character and ethical standards, but which he might equally choose to abuse.

When people choose their doctors for themselves, they face the danger of making a mistake, of being misled by superficial qualities such as a smooth tongue, a polished manner, an expensive suit, a tastefully furnished suite of rooms, excessive confidence and even boastfulness. But it is by no means certain that a lack of choice such as prevails in the British system will preserve them from scoundrels either. It is true that, where commercial gain is possible and permissible, charlatans are more likely to arise. But it is also true that the hope of commercial gain is a powerful incentive to genuine inventiveness and innovation. It is unlikely that you can have the advantage without the disadvantage; and it is no accident that American medicine has been by far the most inventive in the world, at least for the past half-century.

As we have seen, he who pays the piper eventually comes to call the tune; and where the paymaster is a bureaucracy, the tune will be such as pleases bureaucracies. The standardisation of medical care is already well under way, standardisation being something that bureaucracies both understand and desire. The process gives them power, and the need to keep it going justifies their existence. Bureaucracies are comfortable with the average, with the mean (which is not always golden); they also have a preference for the cheap. What they cannot measure does not count for them, or even fails in their estimation to exist. They will always demand standards that approximate to the mean performance. The process of reducing everything to the average will, perhaps, eliminate the dreadful; but it will also eliminate the excellent, the flamboyant and the imaginative. And in the long run, the excellent exerts more of an influence on medical practice than the dreadful. What begins as a startling innovation in a specialised centre gradually becomes normal practice elsewhere, so that procedures and treatments that once amazed the world are soon available (without the need for any central direction) in sleepy little district hospitals far from the centres of scientific advance.

Bureaucracies do not understand the idea of creative failure. If bureaucracies had ruled medicine at the beginning of the era of open heart surgery, no such surgery would be performed today, since initial assays were expensive failures. Cost-benefit analysis of the type beloved of bureaucracies would have prevented the development of heart transplants, since the extra few days of life that the first such transplants conferred were far too dearly bought. There are always pressing needs to be met that will take precedence over innovation if cost-benefit analysis is employed as the only decision-making instrument. One is reminded of the kind of people who see in the cultural monuments of the past only mute testimony to injustice and waste: why did people build palaces, paint pictures, construct fine furniture, write literature, pursue abstruse scholarship, when all around them there was poverty and starvation that could have been alleviated by their efforts, had they abandoned their luxurious pursuits? Cost-benefit analysis would never have permitted the construction of the Pyramids or Chartres Cathedral, though the world would undoubtedly have been a poorer place without them. If it had been left to the bureaucrats, Man would still be in the caves; their effect upon medicine will be no more creative.

The preservation of the independence of the medical profession is therefore a matter of the utmost moment. It is the only way, in the long run, that patients and doctors can maintain a genuinely personal and therapeutic relationship. It is the only way the morale of the medical profession can be sustained: and who wants to be treated by demoralised doctors? It is the only way that the impetus towards technical progress will continue.

And the only way for the independence of the medical profession to be maintained is for the funding of healthcare to be decentralised, so that there is no single piper who calls the tune. The more pipers there are, the more independent it will be.

Of course, independence brings with it the duty of self-regulation. It has been suggested – in Britain at least – that attempts at self-regulation by doctors in the recent past have not been very effective: there have been several well-publicised scandals. There have been incompetent doctors, lecherous doctors, arrogant doctors and even murderous doctors. The government has all too eagerly latched on to these stories, for two reasons: first, it wishes to divert public attention from the manifold deficiencies of the country's health services, which have nothing to do with the deficiencies of doctors, but which would require genuine political and moral courage to put right; and second, because it does not really believe in self-regulation anyway, not merely of doctors but of anyone else. It believes in perfection by regulation, which – by coincidence – grants it a providential role in society.

Once again, a judgement is made by reference to an impossible standard: in this case of a medical profession, with a hundred thousand members, in which there are no villains, no lechers, no exploiters, no incompetents, no criminals, no psychopaths. The system of regulation is judged by the standard of a system so perfect that every deviation from high standards is at once noticed and appropriate action taken. The ideal regulators have complete insight, of course, not only into what has happened but into what will happen: they will be able to predict with complete certainty which doctor will turn out to be a rotter if left to his own devices. And when such a system is in place, there will be no more scandals, no more bad or wicked doctors, every doctor will be superbly competent, and so forth.

This medical paradise, where everything will be for the best, will be brought about by constant form-filling, which will occupy at least a fifth of the doctor's working hours. He will be treated as guilty until he can prove himself innocent – for the next few months, when the whole inquisitorial process will begin again. Doctors will rue the day they were born, or at least the day they qualified.

The demand for perfection in the healthcare system is fundamentally childish, given the acknowledged imperfections of Man. It is the demand that life be emptied of risk or untoward events.

3

The Promethean Bargain:
Imposing Limits on Medicine

Many doctors practise for many years without encountering a moral dilemma. This is not because they are morally obtuse: it is because their work is straightforward and uncontroversial. Patients come to them and they attempt to cure, or at least to comfort, them. A surgeon is not tortured by doubts as to whether it is morally right to cut out an appendix, though he might sometimes be in doubt about the accuracy of his diagnosis.

Still, moral dilemmas do arise in medical practice, and more frequently than they used to. One recent example from my own experience: an elderly man suffering from both dementia and a form of cancer was sent to me for my opinion as to his mental competence to give or withhold his consent to a long and complex operation, which would last several hours, and which would, on the balance of probabilities, prolong his life by six to twelve months. His relatives, who were, in my estimation, more genuinely interested in his welfare than in any legacy (something that in such situations is by no means to be taken for granted), were much opposed to the operation – but their opinion had no legal standing. They said that the ill man was but a shadow of his former self: and while he still enjoyed his food and a pint of beer, he spent most of the day dozing in his armchair, only to wander about at night in a confused and disorientated fashion. Once or twice he had failed even to recognise his own wife of more than forty years.

I decided in the end that the man did not have the mental capacity to decide for himself whether or not to have the operation. If a question was put to him directly, he might give an answer that appeared sensible enough, the result of a process of reasoning. If asked 'Do you want an operation that will last several hours and that will prolong your life by up to a year?' he would reply, 'Yes.' But he appeared to me to be replying more to a tone of voice than to a complex question. If I asked him, 'Do you want an operation lasting several hours that might not work and which means you will have to stay in hospital for three weeks afterwards to recover from it?' he would reply, 'No.' And if I asked him immediately afterwards what I had just asked him, he would be quite unable to say. He knew he had cancer, but was under the impression that a previous operation had cured him. It seemed to me that any consent he gave or withheld could hardly be said to have been given in an informed way. Even if at any given moment he truly grasped the import of what he was being told or asked, his grasp would have slipped a few moments later: so that a consent that might have been valid at the moment it was given could not be considered valid a moment afterwards. Its validity was at best momentary and fleeting.

Of course, the concept of informed consent is pretty slippery. How informed is informed? Does every last possibility or complication have to be discussed with a patient before he can be said to have made an informed choice? The amount of information available on any medical procedure or medicament is, if not infinite, at least very large: so large, in fact, that even the world's greatest expert on it may not know it all. It is not only the patient, therefore, who is uninformed: it is his doctor as well. In a sense, all human action sets sail on a sea of ignorance. Was it not the greatest discoverer in the history of humanity, Sir Isaac Newton, who said that he had played with some smooth pebbles or pretty shells on the seashore, while all before him lay the ocean of truth waiting to be discovered? But ignorance, like knowledge, is relative, and the need for action imperative. We all have to do the best we can in the circumstances.

When I was a student, I worked for a time for a surgeon of great renown, honoured nationally and internationally. He was a man in every way admirable. An excellent technician, he had advanced the science of surgery by his researches. He was unfailingly polite and kind to his subordinates and to students, even those who did not meet his high expectations of them. But what I, who never intended to be a surgeon, most admired in him was his manner of dealing with his patients. He was the opposite of the gruff but expansive and egotistical surgeon of popular imagination (and who used really to exist), who throws tantrums in the operating theatre and walks round the ward barking 'Leg off tomorrow!' from the end of the bed, striking fear into the hearts of the patient and the staff alike. On the contrary: like a man with perfect musical pitch, he was able to adapt his explanations and recommendations to the level of understanding of his individual patients. He did not tell them all the same thing, but estimated – with unfailing accuracy, it seemed to me – not only their intellectual but also their emotional capacity to absorb and utilise information. He was not a one-size-fits-all man, and probably did not have in his mind an unfailing ethical principle to guide him, such as, for example, 'The patient has a right to information about his condition and treatment so that he can make an informed choice'. Rather, he was actuated by genuinely humane feelings and thoughts, combined with rough but nevertheless binding ethical intuitions. And he was clearly a paternalist, in the sense of acknowledging his own inescapable duty to estimate what was in his patient's best interests to know. The fact that he must sometimes have made a mistake (because we humans are fallen creatures) did not deter him or turn him from his path. Of the benefits of this non-egotistical paternalism I shall have more to say later.

But to return to my cancer patient. Having decided that he was not able to make a meaningful decision for himself, it became incumbent upon the doctors – both legally and ethically – to act in the man's best interests. But what were they, and how were they to be ascertained? Was a prolonged existence regardless of its quality and content in his best interests or not? His relatives certainly thought not: but the law accorded them no special standing in the determination. The law required that the question be answered as if the patient were an atom vibrating in the ether.

There is no judgement more dangerous than that someone else's life is not worth living. The passing of this judgement can all too easily become a habit: for it gives the person passing it an intoxicating sense of power. An intellectual might think that the unexamined life is not worth living: in which case he would happily dispense with the lives of the majority of people on earth. The enjoyment of a beer a day can make life worth living; and even those who seem by temperament incapable of enjoying themselves even to this extent are not generally anxious to die prematurely. The decision to stay alive or to commit suicide is seldom made as if it were a problem in double-entry bookkeeping, with pleasures on one side of the balance sheet and pains on the other, leaving a plus or minus balance in the end that determines whether one puts one's head in the gas oven or goes back to work tomorrow morning.

Some ethicists have argued that, in a case like the one with which I was presented, the question should be decided on the basis of what the person would have wanted for himself before his incapacity declared itself. But this is open to two objections: first, it usually cannot be known for certain what a person would have wanted for himself, and second (as we have already seen), what a person wants for himself is likely to change as his circumstances change. Most people do not sit about speculating upon what they would like in the event of the circumstances that will, unbeknown to them, actually arise. It is likely, but not certain, that a university professor would find the prospect of the dissolution of his intellectual faculties more alarming than a footballer would: but it does not in the least follow that the professor would wish to die sooner than the footballer.

In the case in question, I decided that it would be wrong for the man to have the palliative operation: or rather, that it would be better if he did not have it. My decision was based more upon a gestalt of the whole situation than on an ethical algorithm of the kind that is supposed to lead to an indubitable and indisputable answer. (I have generally found that when people of a philosophical cast of mind, who want to have all decisions firmly based upon first principles, come to a repellent conclusion, having argued from those principles, they do not question the argument, as most unphilosophical people would, but accept their reasoning and their conclusion *in toto*, and claim they would be happy to see their repellent conclusions move from the realm of theory into that of practice. I am not sure what proportion of all the philosophers, who are of course increasingly numerous, who argue in favour of the permissibility, desirability or even obligatory nature of euthanasia, whether voluntary or involuntary, would be willing personally to administer the *coup de grâce* to Granny upstairs: nor am I sure whether I should prefer a philosopher who would be willing to one who would delegate the task to someone else. In this connection, it is a pleasure to acknowledge the courage with which Dr Kevorkian, popularly known as Dr Death, and inventor of the Mercitron that has brought easeful death to quite a number of people who had nothing wrong with them, has aligned his practice with his principles: though it seems to me that anyone with even minimal psychological insight would, on reading his memoirs, entertain doubts as to his motives. A man who spends much of his life campaigning, as Dr Kevorkian campaigned, for the use of condemned prisoners as subjects for physiological experimentation, on the grounds that it is a shame to waste the opportunity, and even for the establishment of an entire special branch of medicine devoted to such experimentation, must be, well, odd. Dr Kevorkian is the perfect example of a man who follows an argument to its logical conclusion, and then fails to understand that there must be something wrong with the argument.)

I thought it best that the man with both dementia and cancer should not be subjected to the ordeal of an operation and convalescence because it would prolong his life by only a comparatively short period; because, during a previous stay in hospital, he had become increasingly confused, distressed, agitated, aggressive and anxious to leave, so that he was prepared to fight his way out; because the period he would have to spend in hospital after his operation was not negligible by comparison with the period by which his life would be prolonged; because the operation was uncertain to be successful in any case; because the quality of his life during its prolongation by the operation was unlikely to be high, and would almost certainly deteriorate further; and because his relatives, who knew him best and appeared to have his interests at heart, and who would would have to look after him once he was discharged from hospital, were opposed to it, thinking it cruel, pointless and meddlesome, even though they acknowledged that the decision was not theirs finally to take.

If any of these factors had been different I might have come to a very different conclusion. If the patient had shown clear signs of enjoying life thoroughly; or if the operation would almost certainly have prolonged his life by five years or more; or if his relatives had been strongly of the opinion that the operation should be performed, come what may, and had been prepared to take the consequences: then I might have recommended differently. Legally speaking, the last factor should not have weighed at all: except that, in seeking and acting in the patient's best interests, the doctor surely has to consider the patient's social circumstances, because no man is an island. Or if he is an island, his interests are very different from those of someone is not.

The case illustrates the fact that it is very difficult to reduce medical ethics to a few simple principles, which can then be applied to any situation that arises. Such general principles as

universally apply are so banal as to be worthless. Of course the
doctor should act with benevolence rather than malevolence;
of course he should strive to do good rather than harm. But
does anyone over the age of six need to be told this? I
remember as a child of that age the visits to our house of our
family doctor when I had mumps or tonsillitis. He made little
jokes of the kind that I was then able to understand, at the
same time peering down my throat through his gold-rimmed
half-moon spectacles. I was reassured by his air of omniscience
and omnicompetence. He was to me the model of perfect
human benevolence, and it did not occur to me for a moment
that he might be anything else. I did not even at that age have
to be told that a doctor should be benevolent rather than
malevolent.

And if a doctor were to act malevolently (with regard to his
patients, I mean, not in his private life), would he be likely to
change his ways on being reminded of this overriding ethical
principle? Would Dr Shipman, the general practitioner in
Hyde, Cheshire, who murdered an as yet uncertain, but very
large, number of his elderly patients, have been brought up
short by being reminded of the principle of benevolence and
non-malevolence? Would he, in the midst of his murderous
career, suddenly have said to himself, on being informed of this
principle, 'I see now that what I have been doing is wrong, and
therefore I really must stop it?'

Two concepts are now fashionable in medical ethics, that of
personhood and that of personal autonomy. I do not find either
of them very helpful. At least one of them, personhood, has
sinister implications.

I think that most medical ethicists (a profession brought
into being by the increased technical powers and possibilities
of modern medicine) argue backwards from a conclusion that
they wish to reach. They invent concepts and premises that,
with the help of a few syllogisms, will establish their favoured
conclusions: in other words, they present reasoning backwards
as if it had been reasoning forwards, so that what appears like

rationality is actually rationalisation. No doubt we all do this sometimes in our moral argumentation, often to justify acts we have performed that we know in our hearts to be wrong or dishonourable: indeed, there is a good case to be made for saying that this is the predominant form of human reasoning about morals. In many people, moral reflection is but the search for good reasons for bad deeds; and in the fastness of his prison cell, perhaps even Dr Shipman is busy constructing arguments as to why it was right and proper of him to have dispatched so many victims.

What, then, are the conclusions that the concepts of person-hood and personal autonomy are intended to support, justify, and even make intellectually inescapable? Among others, that both abortion and euthanasia are permissible.

Opponents of abortion believe that the embryo is 'ensouled' at the moment of fertilisation. It follows from this that the embryo and later the foetus is worthy of exactly the same moral consideration as a human being that has been born. Deliberately to kill a human embryo is therefore to murder as surely as to gun a man down in the street. I do not believe it.

Consider the following theoretical possibility. A pregnant woman suffers from an illness from which she will die unless she has an abortion. Is it permissible for her to have it?

Hardly anyone would say that it was not. The reason for this is simple: it is better to have only one death than two, and abortion represents the only practical way in this situation of saving a life. One does not here abort to kill the foetus: one aborts to save the life of the mother.

Whether it is permissible to kill one person to save the life of another is, of course, itself a far from simple question. If a bandit is holding someone hostage, and plausibly threatening to kill him, it might be necessary to shoot him dead to save the hostage's life. The information upon which the hostage's saviour must act will almost certainly be less full than that upon which the doctor who decides to end a woman's preg-nancy must act; and it might even emerge after the bandit has been killed that he had neither the means nor the intention of killing his hostage. Still, not many people would shed tears over his fate, even so.

What this situation clearly demonstrates, however, is that we do not truly believe that one human life invariably is of equal worth to another. If we did, it would be a matter of indifference to us whether the hostage or the hostage-taker was killed: but it is not.

Of course, the foetus in the mother who will die if her pregnancy continues is not to be compared morally to the hostage-taker (though to hear some extreme feminists talk, you might think it was). Unlike the bandit, the foetus has no conscious intentions, either good or bad. But we have already seen that in certain circumstances we do not attribute equal worth to all human lives: therefore, even if we were to attribute full human life to the foetus (or, *a fortiori*, to the embryo), we should still not be obliged to view its life as being of equal worth to that of the mother.

In fact, no one truly feels that a foetus of, say, nine weeks' gestation is a human being in quite the same way as a child of nine years. Many pregnancies end spontaneously in an abortion (that is to say, a miscarriage); but if a woman who had had such a spontaneous abortion were to mourn the conceptus in precisely the same way, and with the same intensity, as she would mourn the death of a nine-year-old child, we should soon regard her as either mentally ill, or as overwrought and self-indulgent. Emotions should be (more or less) proportionate to the events that give rise to them.

The moral equivalence of a foetus and a fully fledged human being is a fiction. Sometimes, as we shall see, moral fictions are necessary; but this is not one such occasion.

Let us try a little thought experiment. Suppose there were a woman who would die if her pregnancy were brought to term, but whose child, if she were allowed to die, could be saved. (It should be remembered that, for much of human history, such were the dangers of childbirth that, statistically speaking, almost any termination of pregnancy was much safer than any childbirth.) Would it be permissible to perform an abortion on her? Or would it be right to demand of her that she carry her pregnancy to term, that her child might live, thereby saving more years of human life than if her own life were to be saved? Surely abortion would still be permissible: for while it might be a noble thing for someone to lay down his life for another, it cannot actually be required of him as an obligation. Indeed, if it could be so demanded, the nobility of the deed would be lost.

Again this thought experiment demonstrates that we do not consider the life of the mother and that of her unborn child to be strictly equivalent, as being worthy of precisely the same moral consideration.

The arguments against abortion, on the ground that the embryo or the foetus is fully human and therefore cannot under any circumstances be killed, fail: for more than one reason.

But what of the arguments advanced by those who not only believe that abortion is permissible, but seem enthusiastically to favour it? I do not think their arguments are very much better either: and as for their enthusiasm, I find there is something distasteful about it.

They argue as follows: first that an embryo or foetus does not have the qualities of personhood that would entitle it to full moral consideration; and second that respect for the personal autonomy of the pregnant woman entitles her to decide for herself whether she carries the pregnancy to term or not.

Personhood is not easy to define. It is a question of having conscious goals, plans and directions in life, self-generated, which form a pattern in life. A person has a biography, not just a past. In this sense, an embryo or foetus is clearly not possessed of the qualities of personhood, any more than is a newt or a fish. Unfortunately, neither is a one-month-old baby. So if it is permissible to kill a foetus because it has not the attributes of personhood, it is permissible to kill a one-month-old baby for the same reason. Indeed, it would be permissible to kill a surprising proportion of the human race on such grounds. Not only would infanticide be an option for disenchanted parents, but so would the elimination of the mentally handicapped. Then there are the chronically or incurably mentally ill, whose fate under the dispensation of personhood would not necessarily be a happy one. And there are the demented also, who do not seem any longer to possess the attributes, whatever they might be, of personhood. Of the many people who, though of normal intelligence, never quite reach the heights of personhood demanded by the philosophers, I shall not speak. But if anybody thinks I exaggerate, I refer them to the work of Professor Singer, the Australian philosopher, now at Princeton, who – though Jewish – was unable to see on a lecture tour of Germany why his endorsement of euthanasia might cause some anger there.

What is morally permissible has a tendency to become – thanks to the doctrine of rights, and to the ever-more rigorous arguments of moral philosophers – compulsory.

Of course, it might be objected that it is impermissible to kill a baby because it has the potential for personhood. But so, by the same token, has an embryo or a foetus. If the potential for personhood is to count as a barrier to killing, then abortion is impermissible.

It is not as if no practical attempt had ever been made before to distinguish between forms of human life that had a right to continued existence and those that did not. The Holocaust, in fact, had a full rehearsal in Germany: the elimination of the mentally ill, as being 'life unworthy of life'.

The concept of personhood, though it pretends to intellectual rigour, reintroduces all the problems of deciding when an embryo or foetus becomes 'ensouled'. At what point does a living being become endowed with personhood? Is such a being entitled to no protection against would-be death-dealers until such time as it becomes 'personificated'? It is, in fact, impossible to state at what precise moment in his life a human becomes fully self-conscious and therefore a person in the philosophers' sense, with plans and projects of his own choosing. There is a famous letter by Chekhov, written to his brother, in which he states that he woke up one fine morning with the realisation that he was a free agent, not a slave, and that he no longer had to kiss the hands of priests, behave obsequiously to relatives, etc., as he had hitherto done. Chekhov was twenty-five when he wrote the letter, which as a literary document is moving and impressive, but which, taken as a literal record of fact, is open to doubt. People grow imperceptibly into themselves; they change as a result of their experiences (that, after all, is what consciousness is for). The concept of personhood is hopelessly vague and inadequate as a criterion for deciding whether a living organism is worthy of the highest moral consideration or not.

What of personal autonomy? It is clear that, as a general rule, a person should be accepted as the best judge of what his own future actions should be. I have refrained from saying his own interests, because long years of medical practice have convinced me that people frequently, perhaps even usually, act against their own interests, insofar as these are objectively ascertainable. (I think it was Dostoyevsky who remarked that if he were the subject of a perfectly benevolent ruler, who acted only for the general and particular good of his subjects, he – Dostoyevsky – would do something against his own interests merely to express and preserve his own freedom and personality. There might be something of this in the repeated refusal of patients to take medical advice, for example to stop smoking, which they know to be both sensible and well meaning. But there are many other reasons why a person may act against his or her own interests, including weakness of will and wilful blindness as to what they actually are. In my own practice, I have seen scores, if not hundreds, of women who return to the men who abuse them, injure them, break their bones, steal their money, half strangle them, drag them by their hair across the room, suspend them by their ankles from high windows, humiliate them in public, threaten them with death, accuse them of infidelity when they themselves have concubines all over the city whom they treat in precisely the same fashion, lock them in rooms or even in cupboards, truss them up with ropes, throw acid in their face, make them walk with their eyes turned towards the ground so that they do not catch sight of other men, refuse them permission to speak to their parents, abandon them only to return when and as they wish, and so forth. The women say they return to these men because they love them, but eventually the worm turns. But why not before? In the course of accepting the abuse, sometimes for years, they self-deceivingly believe obviously insincere expressions of repentance, as well as promises, already broken innumerable times, never to repeat the abuse. They believe in order to persuade themselves of the reasonableness of not leaving. Even worse, such women often do not reflect on their experience in any profound way, once they have left their abuser. They do not ask themselves, for example, whether the abuse they suffered was in any way predictable from the character, conduct and history of the man before they chose to live with him – it usually was. The natural result of this failure to reflect is that, with depressing frequency, the next man they find is of precisely the same type, and the whole sorry cycle begins again. However one chooses to describe this behaviour, it cannot, without violence to the meaning of the words, be called the pursuit of self-interest on the part of the women.

The doctor has to accept that many people sleepwalk their way through life, doing things that are bad for them and failing to do those things that are good for them. He must learn to accept with a good grace the fact that many people will not accept his advice even in theory, let alone put it into practice. Occasionally, but only occasionally, he will overrule their refusal of his treatment. For the most part, he must reconcile himself to the prospect of some of his patients dying, or ruining their lives, through stubbornness, ignorance and weakness of will.

To the extent that he does not (with a few limited exceptions) force his treatment upon people, the doctor accepts the principle of personal autonomy. But this still does not mean that he accepts his patient as being an absolute authority on his own welfare, or on what medical treatment he should have. To do so would be a complete abrogation of the doctor's duty. If a patient comes to him demanding certain drugs or a certain medical procedure that he considers unnecessary or harmful, he does not simply accede to the patient's request because he believes in the patient's right of self-governance, or believes that the patient is necessarily the sole judge of his own best interests. The doctor is not the simple executor of the patient's will.

This is not an unimportant point. Doctors are frequently confronted by patients who have heard of a new drug or treatment that, half-comprehended, they think would be just the thing for them. But just as a parent should know how to say no to its child, so a doctor should know how to say no to a patient. In so doing, he is claiming superior judgement (on this particular subject) to that of his patient. Doctor knows best.

This is not to say, of course, that the doctor's every individual judgement has always been, is and will always be right. Like any other mortal, he makes mistakes. But the choice in human affairs is never between perfection on the one hand and total error on the other. A professional arrangement in which the doctor's judgement is independent of that of his patient serves humanity much better on the whole than an arrangement in which the doctor merely carries out the patient's wishes – or whims. To suggest that the doctor does not, at least very often, know best is to suggest that theoretical knowledge, prolonged training and long experience count for nothing. In other words, it is a position of pure irrationalism.

The relationship of doctor to patient is not that of shop-keeper to customer. The patient does not simply make a choice between the goods on display, though – with the increasing crudity that characterises our social thought these days – it is often suggested that he should. (Recently, for example, the British minister of health said that patients nowadays expected to be treated like customers.) And it is true that Bernard Shaw, nearly a century ago, said that if you paid a man to cut off your leg, he would do so. This, according to Shaw, was a decisive argument in favour of state-funded medicine: forgetting that, if it is really true that he who pays the piper always and without exception calls the tune, state medicine opened up the far more sinister prospect of state-mandated amputations. It was Shaw, of course, who said that all professions are conspiracies against the laity: a silly, shallow dictum, combining technical ignorance, adolescent cocksureness and intellectual dishonesty in equal measure (it was, as they say, no accident that Shaw later became an admirer of both Mussolini and Stalin). It is precisely the professional ethos and ethics of medicine which offer the patient his only guarantee against the flagrant charlatanism and outright exploitation that would otherwise flourish in the healing enterprise. This is so obvious that one would have thought that even a Bernard Shaw could have seen it: but he always preferred a *bon mot* to the truth. And it is no criticism of professionalism that it sometimes fails to protect the public as it is supposed to do. If human institutions are to be criticised and destroyed because they sometimes fail in their purpose, none will be left standing. The only way standards can invariably be met is by having no standards at all.

The doctor cannot, and should not, then, think of his patient as a purely autonomous concatenation of wishes, as many as possible of which should be fulfilled. Among other considerations, the patient is a social being, not an atom of consciousness in a void.

Let us return in the light of these considerations to the question of abortion. We have already seen that it is not absolutely impermissible. Does that mean, then, that is always permissible?

Believers in patient autonomy believe that it is: that abortion on demand represents an advance in human freedom and moral sensibility. A woman, they say, is sovereign of her own body, and therefore has the right to abort a pregnancy for whatever reason she might have, be it serious or trivial. She is the only person who need be consulted in the decision: for she is the only interested party.

Yet jurisdictions in which abortion is permitted at all are agreed that it would be wrong to abort, say, a week before the baby was due. Such late abortion is permitted nowhere. In other words, the pregnant woman is not absolute sovereign of her own body: at least, she loses her sovereignty at some point or other during her pregnancy. Someone else, or society, is deemed as having an interest that transcends hers. The precise moment that this happens is a matter of contention: but that it happens is accepted by all.

A pregnancy is treated by extreme exponents of a woman's right to abortion as if it were the result of parthenogenesis: that is to say, of the division of an ovum without fertilisation into an embryo and then into a foetus. Irrespective of the possibility that parthenogenesis might one day become a technical reality, it remains the case that human pregnancies are not the product of a mother alone. A father is involved. This might seem so obvious that it is not worth remarking upon: except that, in most discussions of the question of abortion, the existence of a foetus's father is ignored altogether, as if it were a moral irrelevance.

There are, of course, circumstances in which the existence of a biological father is morally irrelevant. Perhaps these undesirable circumstances are becoming more frequent, precisely because the importance of the father's contribution to procreation is so often overlooked by moral philosophers. It is only natural – though nonetheless regrettable and wrong – that men should behave irresponsibly in the matter of pregnancy if their contribution to it is so signally disregarded. Where a pregnancy is the result of rape, or where the man abandons the pregnant woman for fear of being asked to make a financial contribution to the child's upkeep (a pattern I have seen repeated on innumerable occasions), it is clear that the father, or impregnator, has no claim on the outcome of the pregnancy.

But in any civilised society, this is not the spirit in which children are conceived. (The fact that this is the spirit in which an increasing proportion of children are conceived in Britain, at least, is a sign of moral retrogression in our civilisation, a civilisation which is, or ought to be, more than the sum of our technical progress.) Two parents decide that they want a child, as an expression both of their love for each other and of life itself, which they want to continue after them. Ideally, the conception of a child is a statement of faith in the goodness of life. The father's part in conception is not negligible, and neither are his responsibilities once the child is born, both to the child and to its mother. The fact that it is in practice difficult to give legal expression to the father's importance does not in the least tend to lessen it.

To speak, therefore, of the conceptus as if it were the mere property of the pregnant mother, to do with or dispose of as she sees fit, as if it were (for example) a piece of unwanted furniture, is staggering in its crudity, and in its failure to reverence or even respect life. It is indicative of a selfish, unsocial, solipsistic world view; of a society of inflamed egos, unable to accept any limitation on the expression of it members' whims. It is not surprising, therefore, to learn of women who have abortions to spite their lovers, or merely to demonstrate the independence of their will. A friend of mine, a doctor, told me of a patient who demanded an abortion because she did not want to be pregnant while she was on holiday in Spain.

This was certainly not what was in the minds of British legislators when they legalised therapeutic abortion in 1968. It was intended as a humane measure to reduce genuine suffering, not to make the question of whether to continue with a pregnancy or not as unimportant as the question of which detergent to take from a supermarket shelf. People who treat the major questions of human existence in this fashion will soon deteriorate in character. But the fact that, within a few years, scores of thousands of abortions were being performed was taken as evidence that there had been a pent-up demand for the procedure all along: the numbers themselves being a tribute to the wisdom and foresight of the legislation.

This fails to recognise that, at least in the modern world, supply often creates its own demand. And what starts out as a privilege, with permission granted in special circumstances, soon becomes a right, at least in the minds of people who want the privilege extended to them. To take the example of abortion once again: the British legislators stipulated that one of the grounds for an abortion to be performed should be that continued pregnancy constituted a threat to the health of the woman. It wasn't long before it was argued that any pregnancy constituted a threat to a woman's health, insofar as the maternal mortality rate, though dramatically lower than in former times, was still higher than the fatality rate when abortion was performed. This wasn't at all what the legislators had meant, of course; they had in mind conditions such as toxaemia of pregnancy, in which a woman might die of hypertensive crisis if the pregnancy were not ended.

But the real escape clause in the legislation was the one that referred to the social or psychological wellbeing of the mother or of her existing children. Again, it isn't very difficult to imagine what the legislators had in mind: they meant circumstances in which, for example, the wife of a brutal husband, who already had four children by him, had been abandoned without financial or emotional support, but was pregnant with a fifth child. Irrespective of whether it would be right to perform an abortion in such circumstances, they were the kind of circumstances the legislators visualised when they framed the law.

Their intentions were soon subverted, however, because they failed to take into account the reflexive nature of all human action. Human suffering and welfare are seldom to be understood by reference to absolute standards. Even in the most extreme of circumstances, for example those of Auschwitz, a person's psychological reactions make a difference to his ability to survive and recover. It is said that those inmates who were possessed of strong beliefs, either political or religious, which gave a framework of meaning to all that befell them (it did not matter whether that framework made sense to anyone else), adapted better to conditions in the camp than those who saw nothing in them but meaningless and arbitrary brutality. Those inmates who were so overcome by the horror of the camp that they lost all interest in their surroundings, the so-called Moslems (Islam meaning submission), soon died.

A world of increased possibilities opens up also a world of increased discontent, where those possibilities are not realised. And when abortion is a legal possibility, not only will a demand for it be created, but any woman who is denied one, on the grounds that her case does not fulfil the criteria laid down by others, will feel aggrieved, the victim of injustice and prejudice. It is simply not true that increased choice – an ever greater panoply of possibilities – leads invariably to greater content-ment, let alone greater happiness. Doctors are now afraid of their patients, and fear to deny them what they believe them-selves entitled to: but always getting what you want is also not the path to happiness.

In summary, therefore, we see that abortion is permissible, but it is not a right, nor is it an expedient to which we should lightly resort. It is permissible because we do not believe a foetus, much less an embryo, is morally speaking the equal of a fully conscious human being. We cannot say at what precise moment the transformation from one to the other takes place, and therefore we need the help of both a legal and a moral fiction to guide us. The fact that they are legal fictions, corre-sponding to no scientific reality, or brute fact of nature, is not a criticism of them: because, without such fictions, we become savages. That fiction is best which sustains our humanity and our civilisation.

Abortion is not a right because rights – themselves moral fictions – do not, with one or two exceptions, sustain our humanity or our civilisation. The extreme individualism that considers a woman the absolute mistress of her body is savage and unsocial, a willing and enthusiastic embrace of the Hobbesian state of nature. At some point, the being that grows inside her must be granted society's protection, for reasons both of humanity and civilisation. In the majority of cases, people other than herself have a legitimate interest (I intend no pun) in the outcome of her pregnancy, for no one is pregnant by masturbation alone.

If abortion is permissible but not a right, when should it be performed? It is in considering the answer to such a question that one realises how blunt an instrument is the law. The outer limits of the permissible can no doubt be laid down: that, for example, abortion must not be undertaken after a certain period of gestation. But it will be quite impossible for the law to lay down all the circumstances in which it is permissible or impermissible, because human circumstances rarely present themselves exactly so as to fit prearranged criteria. One size – or even a small number of sizes – does not fit all.

A subtler form of reflection is needed than the mere decision as to whether present circumstances fit predigested criteria. But in order for such reflection to take place, free of coercion or pressure, it is necessary to have a population that is not convinced that every human choice is a consumer choice, that life is one long trawl through supermarket aisles. And what is true of the question of abortion is true of all serious dilemmas in medical ethics. No simple formulae resolve them all.

At the moment, the only authority that is truly accepted by many people is the authority of desire: it is right, because I want it. Oddly enough, this profoundly utilitarian attitude to life does not notably add to the sum of pleasure (the measure, with pain, of all things), to say nothing of true happiness. From this fact it follows that technical progress will never suffice to produce the good life, though the delusion persists that, if it goes fast or far enough, it will eventually do so. Technical advance can reduce certain concrete forms of suffering, from painful or debilitating diseases, for example; but by giving Man the impression that there is no sphere of his existence about which he has no choice, that life is and should be without limits, it reduces acceptance of intrinsic limitation, which is one of the great pillars of human wisdom and contentment.

We are increasingly Promethean in our outlook. For most of its history, medical endeavour has been concerned straightforwardly to alleviate suffering by fighting disease. There was so much disease about that there was not a need, as there is today, to provide a refined definition of it, since everyone was all too familiar with disease and its consequences. The fact that medicine was for most of its history transparently unable to meet the needs of humanity did not in the least destroy faith in the enterprise: when you're falling into an abyss, a blade of grass will appear like a rescuing rope.

But gradually the role of medicine is changing. One sign of this is that, as everyone becomes healthier, doctors show no sign of being any the less busy. Quite the contrary: although there are more doctors than ever before, relative to the population they serve, they are more frantically occupied than ever before. The trend will continue.

Doctors are no longer expected merely to remove obvious causes of misery and danger, such as typhoid or malaria or cancer. Their tasks have expanded greatly. They not merely relieve pain or save lives, but give people what they want, and technology increasingly enables them to do this. Not long ago, a British couple offered their daughter breast implants as a present for her sixteenth birthday, evidently in the belief that shapely breasts of a certain size were the key to the success and happiness of a young woman's life: and so they proposed that the whole panoply of modern medicine, with its almost risk-free anaesthesia and sophisticated surgical techniques, should be employed as a gift.

No comment is necessary on the parents' somewhat reduced conception of the good life; but it is ironic that at the same time as they should be offering the implants as the key to their daughter's future, there should have been other women seeking redress for the harm that such implants had allegedly done them. The fact that the research upon which they based their claim was of very doubtful validity, the fact that their litigation was more likely to have caused their symptoms than that their symptoms to have caused their litigation, should not obscure the significance of the whole episode: that people increasingly demand surgical procedures as a matter of consumer choice, but without accepting any risk. They have become so accustomed to the safety of everything around them, including medical procedures, that when something goes wrong they assume that it must have been someone's fault: but never, of course, their own.

The science that, of course, threatens most profoundly to turn life into one long shopping expedition is the new genetics. Are our fears exaggerated, or is a Brave New World upon us?

There is no point in worrying about things that will not, because they cannot, happen. There is no doubt that we enjoy tormenting ourselves with the moral and psychological implications of distant technical possibilities, as children enjoy stories that frighten them. On the other hand, the pace of technical development is so fast that what seems like science fiction today might well be surpassed by tomorrow.

It is important to realise that some of the claims of genetics have been considerably oversold. How many times have our newspapers reported the discovery of the gene for this or that complex condition, such as schizophrenia, alcoholism or homosexuality, and even ageing itself, only for the claim to be refuted by those who try to replicate the original results? This failure to replicate the results is never as widely or prominently reported as the original claim, and so the impression is given to the public that more is known that actually is known.

The public has come to believe, indeed, that genes are

destiny. The pendulum of popular belief swings between the belief that heredity is nothing and environment is all to the belief that environment is nothing and heredity is all. At the moment, we are in a period of biological determinism. Human behaviour is increasingly explained by reference to Darwinian theory, though the fact that there is no conceivable behaviour that could not be explained by some arcane analogy with the conduct of crabs or mice suggests that the explanatory power of the theory (with regard to Man) is low. Whether Man behaves with psychopathic selfishness or with great self-sacrifice, whether he riots in a football ground or composes the *Mass in B*, his behaviour is explicable Darwinianly.

Popularising books proving that Man is fundamentally no different from a starfish or a gnu, that human life and society are no different from those of bonobo chimpanzees in the forests of the Congo, sell enormously. The maltreatment of children, for example, has been explained in neo-Darwinian fashion. The observation that biological fathers are much less likely to abuse their children both physically and sexually than are stepfathers to abuse their stepchildren is explained by the fact that biological fathers are concerned for the welfare of their offspring because they bear their genes, while the stepchildren of stepfathers, who do not bear their genes, actually represent a threat to the welfare of the abusing stepfather's own biological offspring (if any) because they compete for scarce resources with those biological offspring. Thus, reducing the chances of his stepchildren's success or even survival represents a good deed as far as the survival of a stepfather's children is concerned.

There are a few salient facts, however, which this explanation appears to overlook. The first is that, while stepfathers are many times more likely to abuse their stepchildren than are biological fathers to abuse their own offspring, the majority of stepfathers do not abuse their stepchildren. The theory does not explain, either, why there should nowadays be so many more stepfathers and stepchildren than there were, say, forty years ago. The change (which in my view is not for the better) has been brought about by a change in the ideological, moral and no doubt legal climate; but this change itself is not explicable by reference to Darwinian theory. And if the selfish gene were quite as selfish as it has been made out to be, it is a miracle that more stepfathers do not go the whole hog, and kill their stepchildren.

Be that as it may, there is a widespread perception that human behaviour and indeed society are totally explicable by Darwinian theory; and since Darwinism is a fundamentally biological doctrine, and since genetics is the fundamental basis of biology, it follows that human behaviour and society are explicable genetically. A renewed interest in the genetics of crime, for example, is one natural result of this belief. That the commission of crime is itself biologically determined is a view that has ebbed and flowed for more than a century: hereditary degeneration was the explanation among students of the question at the end of the nineteenth century, an explanation that profoundly influenced the eugenicists who sterilised a lot of people in the hope of eliminating crime and other forms of depravity. Then there was a reaction against such views, when either behaviourism or psychoanalysis ruled the psychological roost, a reaction reinforced very strongly after the revelations of Nazi atrocities committed in the name of biology. I remember the shock in the 1970s of reading the late Professor Eysenck's book *Crime and Personality*, which claimed that criminality was an hereditary trait: it struck me less as erroneous than as heretical, so completely was I an environmentalist at that stage. Eysenck was a maverick figure, but his views are now all but orthodox, and scholarly volumes are published with titles such as *The Genetics of Crime*, which no longer shock or even raise an eyebrow.

At best, though, genetic explications of criminal behaviour might explain the relative propensity of different individuals to commit crime, rather than the actual decisions to commit it. If this were not so, the fact that rates of criminality vary widely across time and between societies could only be explained by the unlikely hypothesis that populations vary in their genetic make-up with regard to the criminogenic genes. For example, it would have to be argued that the stretches of DNA that predisposed people to steal cars and break into other people's houses had become much more widespread in the British population in the last half-century, for reasons unconnected with the survival of the fittest.

It is in the belief that complex human traits – intelligence, musical and mathematical ability, and so forth – are inherited in a simple genetic fashion that will soon become identifiable by DNA probe that people construct imaginary utopias or dystopias, according to whether they think it a good or a bad thing that parents should be able to specify the qualities of their children in advance, and change them by genetic manipulation. This is a very crude way of conceptualising human life, of course: Man is much more than his genes, and his life is not predetermined in anything like so simple a fashion, if indeed it is predetermined at all. It is true that certain studies have been published on identical twins separated soon after birth (identical twins have precisely the same genetic inheritance, having been derived from the same fertilised ovum) that suggest an astonishing congruence between their tastes, mannerisms, opinions and careers, which allegedly must have been genetic because of the earliness and length of their separation. But such reports should be treated with scepticism, for more than one reason: suffice it to say that the identical twins that I know, though brought up together in more or less identical surroundings, turned out very differently. Perhaps this is just the Dostoyevsky factor: the identical twins, having been brought up to go everywhere together and even to wear the same clothes, rebelled in a desire to express their own individuality, and therefore quite consciously went different ways. If so, however, there could be no more conclusive proof that genes are not destiny, at least not human destiny.

These considerations should be sufficient to lay to rest some of the wilder fears of cloning. Brave New World is not just around the corner, and it never will be. This is not to say that the cloning of human beings is morally permissible, much less that it is desirable, but for reasons other than the fear of a totally regimented society, with its alphas, betas, gammas, deltas and epsilons.

The desire to clone a human being from oneself, besides being based on a fundamental misunderstanding of the likely results (as Heraclitus put it, you do not step into the same river twice), is yet another sign of the egotism of our times. In supposing that the cloned offshoot will resemble him in much the same way as the bud of a coelenterate hydra resembles its originator (parent doesn't seem quite the right word here), the person who wants to clone himself is implying that he is the acme of human perfection, so desirable as a specimen that that there should be at least one more in the world exactly like him. There is, in fact, no legitimate reason why anyone should wish to clone himself (or herself): therefore it should never be done.

Reproductive technology has advanced so far that not only has sex been divorced from procreation, but procreation has been divorced from sex. Gone are the days when the way a child came into the world could be taken for granted, and it could be assumed with a fair degree of statistical accuracy that a child had a mother and a father. With increasing frequency, I meet children whose father was – in a manner of speaking – a syringe.

Technical progress has allowed social and biological boundaries to dissolve and disappear. Women of sixty now have children, as do lesbians who have never had sexual intercourse with a man. Women give birth to children that are not biologically theirs, while children who were born of sperm donor are about to gain the right to know who their masturbatory begetter was. It is hard to see in all this extension of choice anything but incipient disaster.

In vitro fertilisation is a technical triumph, but whether it represents anything more than that may be doubted.

Childlessness is no doubt regrettable for those who want a child, but without the kind of beliefs that make it a disaster for many Africans, it is hardly more than regrettable. The idea that something can be done for it, however, makes it more difficult for people to reconcile themselves to the condition, as they might otherwise do. On the contrary, they come to see in childlessness a complete negation of the meaning of life, instead of finding some other path to meaning. (I meet many old couples who were childless, and while barrenness never ceases to be a matter of regret for them, it has not rendered their lives nugatory.) A problem that is potentially soluble but not solved causes us more grief than a problem that is accepted as insoluble at the outset.

In fact, at least three-quarters of all attempts at in vitro fertilisation fail, usually after an immense expenditure of time, effort and money. The disappointment must be great, greater indeed than if no hope had been offered in the first place. It might be said that this is part of the Promethean bargain of medicine: after all, life-saving procedures in, say, cancer, are rare, but the hope is always there (a mere 5 per cent of lung cancers are operable). The hope of saving one's life, however, is surely of a different order from the hope of having a child – unless one believes, along with the hypothecists of the selfish gene, that the whole purpose of life is to preserve one's DNA. It is an open question whether the technique of in vitro fertilisation has added to or subtracted from the sum of happiness in the world (if such a sum could meaningfully be done). For every one successful case there are three unsuccessful: does one person's joy outweigh three people's bitter disappointment?

A final answer can never be given, because it is possible that techniques will improve as a result of practice, and disappointment, at least on such a scale, become a thing of the past. Certainly, no improvement will take place unless there is practice: but the expectation of universal success will soon enough also lead to a diminution of joy.

The control of reproduction is as yet crude by comparison with the control which, thanks to genetic engineering, is all too easily envisaged. Our present efforts at perfecting our offspring may appear to our descendants in a hundred years' time as the days of rag-and-bottle anaesthesia appear to us: faintly comic, though they were miraculous at the time. For example, every baby born is now screened through a simple blood test for a rare inborn disease called phenylketonuria, from which it would develop severe mental deficiency if it consumed food with a certain amino acid. The elimination of that amino acid from the diet allows the baby to grow and develop normally, and so the test averts a few tragedies every year. This is small beer indeed compared with what is to come.

At the moment, our technology with regard to testing children before or just after birth is largely negative: for example, the presence of a child with Down's syndrome can be predicted from a blood test or from amniocentesis, as can an increasing range of defects and inborn errors of metabolism. But even this knowledge is wholly unequivocal in its effects. It presents parents with a dilemma: whether to continue with the pregnancy or not.

It might appear obvious that a handicapped child is a burden best avoided. Who, after all, would want a handicapped child if he or she could have a normal one? Yet it is not the experience of many parents of handicapped children that they are less lovable or loving than other children, and there are few more moving sights than that of the parent of a loving handicapped child caring for him devotedly. Who has not seen happy outings of handicapped children, cared for by devoted men and women, and who would dare to say that it would have been better had these children never been born? But that is what the message of prenatal testing for deficiencies seems to be.

It is for the individual to decide what burdens he can bear.

Given the pace of technical advance, the day cannot be far off, however, when the qualities of children yet to be born will be positively rather than negatively selected. We will not so much eliminate conceptions with defects as select ones with desirable (or rather desired) qualities. This has long been an aim of mankind, particularly with regard to the sex of its offspring. Even today, I sometimes see patients of Indian origin who have gone to 'healers' who have poisoned them with potions that will ensure a boy child (it is invariably the woman who is asked to take them). More and more physical qualities – colour of eyes, hair, and so forth – will become matters of prenatal choice.

Will this matter, so long as the choice is left up to individual parents rather than to the state? (The state's attempts in the past to produce a race of supermen, as in the Nazi Lebensborn experiment, were not only deeply wicked, but pathetic in their basic ignorance of genetics.) Will it matter that more blue-eyed children are born than brown?

A gross imbalance in the sex ratio of children born could, of course, have serious social – or rather, antisocial – effects. Most societies have traditionally valued male offspring more than female, and in China, when only one child was permitted each couple, the infanticide of female babies became commonplace, and a sexual imbalance resulted. If there were far more boys born than girls, competition among males for the attention of females, already the occasion of considerable violence, could increase greatly. Believers in the ability of the marketplace to rectify all errors and imbalances might argue that, when it becomes clear that as a result of the past choice of parents the life of a boy has become much more difficult than that of a girl, parents will choose to have girls rather than boys. But in the meantime there could be a lot of trouble: for rectification of such an imbalance could take many years.

As we have seen, it is unlikely for technical reasons that offspring could be selected genetically for more complex mental characteristics, such as personality and intelligence. Even so, the prospect of parents choosing even the physical characteristics of their future children is enough to make us shudder, and it is instructive to consider why this should be.

Utilitarianism, such as is now the almost unconscious foundation of our moral thinking, can hardly explain why, except in a very convoluted way. After all, the satisfaction of parents' pre-existing desires about what their children should be like can hardly represent anything other than a net gain in human pleasure. Why, then, would it be wrong?

A recent scandal in Britain can give us a clue by analogy. A Dutch pathologist was appointed to a chair in paediatric pathology in Liverpool. He at once gave orders that every organ of every deceased child was to be preserved, regardless of all other considerations. The little corpses were more or less eviscerated, without their parents' knowledge; but the organs were stored in such a haphazard way that they were subsequently scarcely of any use to science.

The professor was clearly a man of an unusual type. According to the official report into the affair, he was a careless pathologist who did not perform his most elementary duties either competently or conscientiously. His enthusiasm for the storage of organs made him appear like a Professor Frankenstein.

Let us leave aside the fact that the scandal about the stored organs broke at a very convenient moment for the government, to distract public attention from uncomfortable revelations about its own ethical standards. Let us leave aside also the abominable wave of sentimentality about dead children that the scandal unleashed: for the British, of course, have a guilty conscience about their children, who are neglected and disliked by their parents to an extent unknown elsewhere in the world, sentimentality about them being therefore a form of cheap reparation. When all is said and done, there was something profoundly distasteful about the way the professor conducted himself and his department.

There was, naturally enough, a great deal of comment on his behaviour, most of it missing the point entirely. The government minister responsible blamed the paternalism of the medical profession (of the paternalism of the government he had rather less to say). Because the parents of the eviscerated children had not given their permission, the scandal was discussed as if the fundamental fault had been the infringement of their rights, for hardly anyone nowadays can see a problem of this nature without reference to rights.

This was nonsense, of course, and behind the distress of the parents who said they thought they had been burying their child when in fact they were burying their child without its vital organs, one heard the hope of monetary compensation, that universal balm of modern souls: that panacea that makes ill healthy, bad good and unhappy happy.

But the wrong that the professor did (though he acknowledged no wrongdoing at all) had nothing to do with the infringement of anyone's rights. Of course, the fact that he outraged the feelings of the grieving parents made what he did worse, but this was not his fundamental fault. If he had treated the corpses of orphan children with no one to grieve over them as he treated the corpses of children with parents, we should not have said that he had therefore committed no fault. On the contrary, it is a moot point as to whether or not his conduct in such circumstances would have been considered worse rather than better.

He did not infringe rights, and he certainly did not steal or abuse anyone's property. The relationship of a corpse to its nearest living relative is not that of an owner of furniture to his furniture: the latter being objects of which he can dispose in any way that he sees fit. If the professor had obtained the permission of the parents of the dead children to feed their corpses to the animals in the zoo, for example, it would not have been permissible therefore for him to have done so. The nearest relatives of the deceased are usually consulted over the disposal of a body, not because they have rights over it, but because elementary human decency demands it.

Neither the state nor the attendant doctor owns a body, for the simple reason that bodies are not objects of ownership in any normal fashion. There is in the relationship of a corpse to society a delicate fabric of considerations, in which now one, now another, might take precedence.

It follows, of course, that the question of informed consent about the use of tissues and organs taken from bodies after death – insisted upon by the British minister of health in the wake of the scandal – is almost completely irrelevant. If no one owns a body, therefore no one gives or withholds consent to use parts of it. In certain circumstances, it is true, the state has the right and even the duty to treat the body as if it owned it: where, for example, foul play is suspected and the matter has to be investigated for the sake of public safety. Then the state acts irrespective of the wishes of the nearest relatives. But even in these circumstances, the state does not truly own the body whose cause of death it is investigating.

In more normal circumstances, the wishes of the nearest relatives are not overridden because there is no pressing need or reason to do so. But the idea that informed consent by relatives to every last act performed by a pathologist at a post-mortem should be sought, in order that there should never be another scandal such as the one at Liverpool, is, of course, absurd for more than one reason.

First, it would not in practice prevent a really determined professor from doing what was done at Liverpool, unless there was in place a system of checking so cumbersome that it would bring the work of all pathology departments to a virtual halt.

Second, it would be impossible to obtain in advance informed consent that did not rely on the pathologist's judgement and discretion, as the pathologist cannot say in advance what he is going to find and therefore what he will need to keep and preserve: to say nothing of the interests of medical science, which might be served by preserving tissue for future research. (The search for the origin of the AIDS epidemic has been much advanced by the preservation of tissue from forty and fifty years ago, whose value to a much later period the preservers could not have anticipated in any detail.) Medical research has a legitimate interest in the disposal of bodies and their parts, but like all other interests, it is not an ace of trumps.

Any genuine system of informed consent (even supposing that such a system were morally desirable) would necessarily be so cumbersome that little pathological investigation would be possible, for the pathologist would have to spend most of his time running back and forth between laboratory and nearest relative, seeking ever more permissions to do ever more tests. And that would be detrimental to humanity: for the clinico-pathological method is one of the pillars of scientific medicine, and is one of the great cultural achievements of Mankind, despite its aesthetically less appealing aspects. If physicians learn by mistakes, it is pathology which draws attention to them in the first place.

The Liverpool professor's fault was more like sacrilege than an infringement of human rights. He did what innumerable pathologists before him did (and I hope will do after him): namely, preserved tissues and organs from the bodies of the dead without asking anyone's permission. What distinguished him from them, however, was the unfeeling, almost perverse way in which he did it, at least if the official inquiry is to be believed (which, of course, is not always the case). He appeared to have no respect for the human remains entrusted to him; he treated them with as little reverence as if they were the left-overs of someone else's meal. The fact that they were children's and not adults' remains was not, of course, of the slightest relevance, except to the sentimental.

Whether or not we believe in a transcendent purpose in life, given it by a supreme being, we have to live as if there were something in human life that distinguishes it from all other phenomena in the universe: in other words, something sacred. It is, of course, much easier to take this view if you are reli-gious; but it is necessary even if you are not. We do not own human life: not even our own, let alone that of our children. We are not therefore free to do with it as we will.

It is this failure to treat life as something beyond an instrument for our own pleasure which is offensive about the idea that parents should choose the physical characteristics of their future offspring, in the same spirit as they choose the colour of their car. Not only does it suggest the trivial view that the most important aspect of life, which more or less determines fate, is physical appearance, reduced to a few relatively simple characteristics; it degrades the importance of human life itself.

We need to tread carefully between freedom and obedience: obedience, that is, to a set of rules that transcends our individual wills. In a post-religious age, this is increasingly difficult to do, for it involves the willing suspension of disbelief and even of enquiry into the metaphysical justification of that set of rules. When Moses handed down the tablets of stone engraved by God, and everyone accepted the provenance of injunctions written upon them, the problem was solved. The American Declaration of Independence and the Constitution once acted in the same way, psychologically speaking, in the United States; they were foundational documents whose provenance was guarantor of their wisdom. But time passed, and a small handful of rights became indefinitely many rights. The purpose of the idea of rights changed: whereas once they were supposed to protect the individual against the dictatorship of society, they came to ensure the dictatorship of the individual over society.

The problem for medical ethics in a post-religious age, in which theoretical advances are matched by an increasing technological ability to interfere with the basic processes of life, is to find some transcendent code to help us decide what is permissible and what is impermissible. Two hundred years ago, Edmund Burke famously remarked that 'men are qualified for civil liberty in exact proportion to their disposition to put moral chains upon their appetites'. But where are the chains to come from, if not from a jealous God prepared to punish transgressors? Burke went on, 'Society cannot exist unless a controlling power upon will or appetite be placed somewhere, and the less of it there is within, the more there is without. It is ordained in the eternal constitution of things that men of intemperate minds cannot be free.'

To an extent, our increased power of control over nature makes us all men of intemperate minds. We do not easily accept limitations on our own appetites. If something is feasible, we feel it ought to be done or, even worse, that we have a right to have it done. Because it might soon be possible for a seventy-five-year-old woman to give birth, someone somewhere will make it happen. And then natural justice will demand that what was permissible in one place and on one occasion must be permissible in other places on other occasions.

It is part of the glory of Man that he sets no limits to his understanding and to his power; but it is also part of his misery. The interplay of ambition and resignation is, or should be, a subtle one. Fatalism in the face of the remediable is wrong; but it is also necessary to know what is worth remedying.

4

A Pill for Every Ill:
Disease and Delusion

The medieval doctor and philosopher Moses Maimonides said that he hoped he would never see in his patients anything other than suffering human beings: a noble aspiration, no doubt, but one that was perhaps easier to satisfy in days when even a minor complaint might all too easily lead to swift death.

More recently, there has been much lamentation over what has been called the medicalisation of life. In 1975, the theologian, historian and anarchist philosopher Ivan Illich began a book that was for a time the bible of the disaffected – *Medical Nemesis*, later republished in expanded form as *Limits to Medicine*, with the ringing words: 'The medical establishment has become a major threat to health. Dependence on professional healthcare affects all social relations. In rich countries medical colonization has reached sickening proportions; poor countries are quickly following suit.'

Illich was both right and wrong. Since 1975, the health of Western populations has continued to improve, despite the threat allegedly posed to it by the medical establishment. People not only live longer, but live more healthily. In Britain in 1975, geriatricians were responsible for the hospital care of patients over the age of sixty-five; but so extended has the lifespan become, and so usual survival beyond the biblical three score years and ten, that geriatricians now attend only to patients over the age of seventy-five, and sometimes even those older than that. It would probably be wrong for the practice of medicine to claim all the credit for the improvement:

but it makes Illich's claim, taken in its most literal sense, look pretty silly. Even more startling advances in the general state of the population's health, relatively speaking, have been made in poor countries than in rich: and while it might not be the practice of medicine as such that has caused these startling advances, certainly the understanding of disease – wholly the achievement of the western tradition of scientific medicine, owing nothing, except in the very distant past, to any other tradition – has enabled it to take place.

In his book, Illich pointed out that many patients are ill because of iatrogenic disease: that is to say, diseases caused by the treatments given them by doctors, rather than by endogenous disease processes. It is well known also that dangerous infections sometimes lurk in hospitals: our newspapers love a good flesh-eating bug that causes an outbreak of necrotising fasciitis in a hospital with which to terrify their readers, as the stories of the Brothers Grimm used to terrify children at bedtime. Medicines have side effects, operations go wrong, patients die on the table, occasionally even the wrong leg is amputated, much to the delight of newspapers; by contrast, the story that Mrs Jones – no, a thousand Mrs Joneses – had operations that proceeded satisfactorily and without complications is not news. Illich represents the intellectual end of the market for disaster. As an anarchist, he is so opposed to the division of labour that he does not want to admit that professional medical care may actually save lives in many cases. When he says that '[epidemics] are not modified any more decisively by the rituals performed in medical clinics than by the exorcisms customary at religious shrines', he is guilty of the oldest rhetorical trick in the trade: *suppressio veri* and *suggestio falsi*. Only an egotistical philistine of limited historical imagination (and one, moreover, pretty sure of his own continued good health) could fail to recognise the tremendous liberation from pain and anxiety that modern medical care truly represents: though, of course, Man being what he is, he always finds a new anxiety to replace the old. Still, I had rather be anxious about the allegedly carcinogenic properties of coffee or overhead power cables than about the date of the next epidemic of bubonic plague. Not even the most ardent masochist or religious mortifier of the flesh would opt for the surgical techniques of three hundred years ago compared to those of today. As to Illich's call for 'the individual to heal himself' in contradistinction to submitting himself to 'the medical and para-medical monopoly over hygienic methodology and technology', one wonders what exactly he had in mind: operations on kitchen tables by people who had never so much as carved a goose before?

Still, it would be unfair not to recognise a sense in which what he wrote a quarter of a century ago does not have considerable resonance today. A great deal of life has been medicalised, though not so much because of the imperialism of doctors, as Illich thinks, but because of the demand of patients – the very people whom he believes are desirous and capable of taking over their own healthcare.

Some doctors, though, have undoubtedly fostered the idea that there is almost nothing beyond the powers of medicine, thanks to new technology. A few years ago, the Harvard psychiatrist Peter Kramer wrote a fundamentally silly book called *Listening to Prozac*, in which he suggested that we were entering an age of designer neuropharmacology. He said that many patients who took the drug Prozac (already so much a part of our culture that it appears on the spell-check of my computer) were surprised to discover not only that they recovered from their depression, but were actually better than they had ever been before. They were more confident, less anxious, more ambitious, less prone to self-doubt, more successful with the opposite sex, less bashful, and so forth. I was reminded of the old joke about the man with the injured hand, who asks the surgeon who is about to operate on it whether he will be able to play the piano after the operation. 'Yes,' replies the surgeon. 'That's funny,' says the patient, 'I never could before.'

Dr Kramer suggested that, with the help of an increasing

panoply of drugs, we would be able more or less to design our own personality. You feel you would like to be a little less earnest, with a better sense of humour? Take a bit of x. You would like to be the life and soul of the party, rather than the wallflower nursing a drink in the corner? Take a bit of y. It was a comforting vision, no doubt, for those who would like to change at least the outward show of their personality, but have not the courage, the perseverance or the ability to do so (as how many of us have?). Swallowing a few pills is an easy option: dose your way to happiness and success.

It is complete nonsense, of course, based on a very crude view of what people are and what makes them as they are. For all the technological wizardry of the modern neurosciences, with their extraordinary scanning machines that light up images of the brain in different colours as we think, or hallucinate, or laugh, or do simple sums in our head, the theories of neuropharmacology are not very sophisticated. Drugs like Prozac are thought to act upon at least one of the neurotransmitters – that is to say, the substances that pass on an electrical impulse from one nerve cell to another – by increasing their availability, and no doubt they do in fact do this. Not only does this not exclude the possibility of other actions, but it is often forgotten that there is a 30 per cent placebo response to tablets or capsules of any kind in depression, and that at the most 70 per cent of patients with severe depression (that is to say, cases carefully selected by researchers) improve with Prozac. In other words a mere 40 per cent of genuinely depressed people, meeting the strictest criteria that can be laid down, respond to the drug – which in this respect is not at all superior to the older antidepressant drugs. Far from being a wonder drug, therefore (such as Prontosil, the first sulphonamide, or penicillin, the first true antibiotic, truly were in their day), Prozac represents a minor advance in therapeutics. It has fewer side effects, and is safer in overdose, than the older antidepressants, but these advantages do not represent a real 'breakthrough', except in terms of marketing. Prozac is now the most widely swallowed drug in the world, but it is not universally effective, as we have seen. Its attraction in much of the world is probably its modernity: one is up to date if one takes it.

Nevertheless, the alleged derangements in cerebral serotonin metabolism (serotonin being the neurotransmitter upon which and through which Prozac supposedly acts, when it does act) have almost entered popular culture, so widely have they been touted. 'It's not me, it's my serotonin,' might be the cry of anyone with anything to be ashamed about. Serotonin – or an insufficiency thereof – is the root of all evil.

It is hardly surprising, therefore, that the drug is handed out for almost any form of human unhappiness, discomfort or existential angst. Life is a matter of getting the cerebral chemistry right, and whose job can it be to do this except the doctor's? Truly there is – because in our brilliant new technological age it stands to reason that there must be – a pill for every ill. When, therefore, the pills the doctor prescribes fail to bring about that state of bliss that is every modern man's birthright, who is to blame but the doctor, for not having chosen the right pill in the first place?

There is a convenience for the doctor in his patient's belief, or rather superstition, that there is a pharmacological answer to every form of human misery: that is to say, it enables him to guide, or hustle, the patient out of his room with reasonable expedition. All he has to do to bring the consultation to a successful conclusion is to write a prescription. The patient is happy because the doctor has implicitly accepted thereby that there is something wrong with him, while the doctor is happy not only because the patient will now leave him in peace, at least for a while, but because there is the faint chance that the prescription will actually do the patient good, over and beyond its placebo effect.

A delicate but absurd dance between the doctor and his patient often follows. The patient has come to the doctor complaining of depression. The doctor, in a desultory kind of way, asks why the patient is depressed. The patient claims not to know, because if he is too specific in his answer the whole pretence that there is something medically wrong with him will be given away. If he says, for example, that he is profoundly unhappy because he drinks too much, his business is going bankrupt, his wife is leaving him and his son has taken to drugs, his complaint is likely to sound absurd: for who in such circumstances, except a totally unfeeling man, could be anything other than unhappy?

So the doctor neither seeks, nor does the patient offer, too many confidences. They are playing a game whose rules they both understand but must never enunciate outright. The doctor agrees not to ask too many questions, and the patient agrees not to tell too many lies. In this way the doctor does not have to spend too much time with the patient, and the patient can continue to think that there is something wrong with him that the doctor can, and should, cure him of.

The first prescription fails to work, of course. That was only to be expected, given the inexactitude of science, even nowadays. But there is no need to despair, because there are plenty more drugs to try, thanks to the inventiveness of the drug companies. It was just bad luck that the wrong one was selected first by the doctor. And if at first he didn't succeed, why, he tries, tries again. Given the extensive nature of the modern pharmacopoeia, it is clear that the dance can last a very long time, for months if not years. The inconvenient fact that the patient's life is not conducive to, or even compatible with, a happy existence is never alluded to: for to do so would be to enter the forbidden realm of judgement.

The distinction between psychiatric disorder and ordinary human weakness is, as is that between misfortune and self-infliction, not always easy to make. It is this fact which makes the creeping medicalisation of human distress possible. As a child, I had an uncle who had frittered much of his money away on the horses and the dogs. In those days, his habit was regarded as weakness of will; nowadays he would be regarded as suffering from compulsive gambling, a bona fide illness that appears in the *Diagnostic and Statistical Manual of the American Psychiatric Association*, a compilation viewed with superstitious awe around the world. The method employed by the authors of the *Manual* is fundamentally that used by St Anselm in the ontological argument for the existence of God: if a thing can be defined, it must actually exist. Of course, all that can be defined does not actually appear there: famously, the decision was taken by the compilers to exclude homosexuality from their next edition, and overnight an illness became a way of life. The *Diagnostic and Statistical Manual* reflects the zeitgeist at least as much as it reflects knowledge about illness.

Pathological gambling, as it is known, appears under the section devoted to disorders of impulse control. What are the criteria for making the diagnosis?

- Frequent preoccupation with gambling or with obtaining money to gamble.
- Frequent gambling of larger amounts of money or over a longer period of time than intended.
- A need to increase the size or frequency of bets to achieve the desired excitement.
- Restlessness or irritability if unable to gamble.
- Repeated loss of money by gambling and returning another day to win back losses ('chasing').
- Repeated efforts to reduce or stop gambling.
- Frequent gambling when expected to meet social or occupational obligations.
- Sacrifice of some important social, occupational or recreational activity in order to gamble.
- Continuation of gambling despite inability to pay mounting debts, or despite other significant social, occupational, or legal problems that the person knows to be exacerbated by gambling.

For the diagnosis to be made, says the *Manual*, the patient must exhibit at least four of these: though why it should be four rather than three or five is no doubt an arcane statistical mystery.

Other disorders of impulse control are the setting of fires, repeated shoplifting, and 'intermittent explosive disorder' (known to previous generations as bad temper). I myself suffer from several impulse disorders, among them an uncontrollable urge to write articles for publications that will pay me to do so – I grow anxious and restless if not asked for any period longer than a few days – and a compulsion to enter bookshops, especially second-hand ones, and buy their wares.

Not long ago, I came across an academic book, written by psychologists working in university departments, suggesting that the repeated commission of crime was an addiction, especially a crime such as that of stealing cars. The more neurologically minded of them even provided diagrams of the cerebral mechanisms by which they thought the addiction might be mediated. The extreme excitement of stealing a car was followed by a 'let-down', the misery of which could be alleviated only by stealing another car. In the most literal sense, therefore, adolescent car thieves were in the grip of a compulsion to steal that was beyond their control, an addiction in the truest sense, complete with craving, withdrawal effects, and an escalating need to continue.

It is certainly true that there are many car thieves who have stolen many cars. I met one young man, aged twenty-one, who claimed to have parted 540 vehicles from their owners in about two years. He was caught on one occasion and admitted to having stolen sixty, for the misappropriation of which he received a sentence of six months' detention, of which he served three. In the meantime, he had made approximately £100,000 from his activities, which had done him little good, since he spent it munificently on giving his friends and acquaintances a free run of the local nightclubs. Certainly, he was unlikely to have earned so much money in any other way for, while possessed of native cunning, he was not otherwise possessed of skills of use to a potential employer. It is, however, regarded generally as rather crude and slightly vulgar to refer to the impunity with which so many crimes are committed as having a bearing on the decision of criminals to commit them, something unmentionable in polite society, as of course is the deficiency of the code of morals that might otherwise inhibit them. By contrast, the man who argues that the compulsive car thief cannot help himself, for purely neurological or neurochemical reasons, is always welcome in the salons of the compassionate, for he shows himself understanding of those less fortunately placed than himself. Oddly enough, the neurological or neurochemical explanation of behaviour is never applied to those whose conduct is perfectly acceptable, or to those who feel the compulsion to catch or punish the wrong-doers. They are autonomous human beings who misuse their autonomy out of sheer malice and ill-will.

No one speaks of an irresistible urge to do good or to behave well. Our virtues require no explanation, because they are the true expression of our innermost being. Our vices, being strangers to us, like the bacteria that cause pneumonia, require physiological explanation and need medical attention.

Addiction is a phenomenon in which the limits of medicine are tested. The reality of the phenomenon of addiction can hardly be doubted. To take one obvious and very serious example of its consequences: delirium tremens. When a man who has been drinking to great excess for some period of time stops doing so, perhaps because of admission to hospital for an operation, or because of imprisonment, he may start to experience vivid visual hallucinations between twenty-four and forty-eight hours later (as well as other familiar withdrawal effects, such as sweating, tremor and epileptic fits), such that he tries to jump out of a window to escape the pursuing chimeras. I have known several such cases, ending with broken legs, fractured spines and so forth. People can collapse and die in delirium tremens: the DTs are a medical emergency. Moreover, a syndrome very similar to DTs sometimes afflicts those who have been taking benzodiazepine tranquillisers (most famously Valium or diazepam, once known as mother's little helpers) for a prolonged period and have suddenly stopped. Dangerous withdrawal effects are also possible after prolonged use of barbiturate drugs, though these are now prescribed far less frequently, if at all, than in days gone by. Curiously enough, the withdrawal effects from prolonged consumption of opiates, regarded by the general public as being the most serious of all, are trivial by comparison. I shall suggest reasons for this widespread and popular misconception later.

Addiction as a physiological phenomenon is real enough, then. But it does not follow from this that it is an illness in any straightforward sense. The disease concept of alcoholism, for example, is profoundly misleading. That excessive drinking can (and often does) lead to physical illnesses in the most literal sense is so well known that it hardly needs saying. The drunk suffers from demonstrable gastritis; his brain rots to the point of dementia; his pancreas packs up and he becomes diabetic as a result; his liver grows fatty, hardens, and becomes cirrhotic; little varices form at the bottom of his oesophagus and eventually burst, so that he dies of exsanguination; and so forth. All this is beyond dispute. But to argue that therefore the drinking that produces these dire results is itself a disease is wrong. It is like arguing that the football that inevitably results in ruptured cruciate ligaments and torn menisci is a disease.

The reality of addiction does not make the addict the helpless cipher, the plaything of his addiction, that is all too often depicted in popular literature and film. If this were the case, no addict would ever successfully have overcome his addiction, but the world is in fact full of former addicts who have thrown down their fags, forsworn the bottle, abandoned their needles, and so forth. And although an organisation like Alcoholics Anonymous believes that alcoholics suffer from a disease, namely alcoholism, it is surely a very odd disease indeed that can be cured (or at least held in abeyance) by the sole exercise of faith and willpower of the kind that AA itself recommends – indeed, that can be cured or held in abeyance only by such faith and willpower. (Not that I have the least desire to denigrate Alcoholics Anonymous. The good that it does is incompatible with intellectual scepticism about the claims it makes; and so great is the misery caused by alcoholism, both to the person who is alcoholic and to the people around him, that it seems to me that an ounce of success in stopping people from drinking too heavily is worth a pound of doctrinal truth on the matter of heavy drinking. In other words, I would have no hesitation in sending a patient to AA, even though I do not subscribe myself to some of the organisation's beliefs. Sometimes truth is not the only or most important value.)

There is no addiction so strong that it cannot be overcome by people taking thought: but whether they do so or not is another matter entirely. Heroin addicts are, like Gaul, divided into three: those who give up, those who continue for many years, and those who die as a result of their rather unattractive practices. If an addict believes that addiction is something so strong that it cannot be overcome by anyone, let alone by him, he is far more likely to belong to one of the latter two groups than the former group, just as a person who suffers from chronic fatigue syndrome (that neurasthenia of the twentieth century) and believes that it is caused by the long-term effects of a viral infection is far less likely ever to recover from it than those who are agnostic as to its causation.

Let us consider some of the complexities of addiction. The addict is inclined to believe that he is in the grip of something that transcends himself, an illness that comes to him from the exterior (and, in this context, his genes are exterior to himself, if he considers his problem to be of genetic origin). Several alcoholics have said to me, in describing and explaining their descent on the social scale, 'And then the beer went mad,' as if the beer drank them rather than they drank the beer.

The addict, then, presents himself to the doctor as a person with no choice but to continue in his self-destructive and antisocial conduct. He has a bona fide medical problem, which it is the doctor's function and duty to solve. This, of course, has the great advantage that, when the doctor fails to solve it, the 'sufferer' (who may actually suffer, but also derives gratification from his consumption of whatever it is he is addicted to) can continue with his habit undisturbed by the thought that he is weak willed or worse.

Now it has been shown experimentally that the way in which addicts – particularly opiate addicts – present themselves to the doctor (or to the social worker, the judge, the probation officer, etc.) is very different from the way in which they present themselves to each other. To the doctor and others who are supposed to 'help' them, they emphasise the horrors of withdrawal, the pangs of craving, and suchlike. This is to underscore the extreme difficulty of giving up, at least without expert help (which they know to be less than expert, because most of them have tried it before and because in any case no one is an expert in another man's willpower). To each other, they emphasise such matters as the best or cheapest source of supply, how best to achieve the greatest desired effect of the drug, and so on. I am undecided whether this duality amounts to conscious dishonesty, but it undoubtedly exists. (When criminals decide to end their careers – as most eventually do – they often come to me in the prison where I work and beg to be moved away from their present company, usually of younger men, who both boast of their criminal exploits and excuse their actions at the same time, using precisely the same dishonest excuses that the reforming criminal once used. He cannot bear any longer to listen to this poisonous mixture of self-congratulation and self-pity.)

In some cases, of course, the addict is genuinely frightened of withdrawal effects. This applies mainly to opiate addicts, and never to alcoholics who have good reason to be frightened of them. The fear of the opiate addict is not so much of the unknown – he may well have withdrawn before – but of the mythology that has grown up around withdrawal. He has been led to believe that withdrawal is a terrible trial that no normal person could be expected to endure: a very convenient belief, insofar as it permits the addict to continue his habit without thinking badly of himself. And society in general has all too easily believed this view of withdrawal from opiates for reasons of its own. In the first place, it helps to explain why it is that so many addicts remain on the drug, despite the ostensible disadvantages of doing so. People who are not themselves addicted are excused from looking any further at why people choose to remain on the drug, or too closely at the lives of addicts, which would tell us some very uncomfortable things about the society we live in. The fear of withdrawal effects conveniently explains all. La Rochefoucauld said that neither the sun nor death can be looked at for very long: and the same applies, as far as the middle classes are concerned, to the lives of drug addicts.

In the second place, the doctrine of withdrawal effects (if I may so call it) is a useful plank in the programme of the progressive demoralisation of life that has long been the aim of the intelligentsia, ever since it revolted against Victorianism and its too-rigid and intolerant set of values. The alleged severity of withdrawal effects, which nobody has a right to demand another person to undergo, excuses the drug addict, and turns a moral problem into a physiological one, which it is the duty of scientists to solve. If a man commits a crime in pursuit of money 'to feed my habit', as the argot puts it, then he is not truly guilty of the crime. It was, as they say, the drugs, not the man.

Perhaps this explains why no one objected to the scene in the commercially successful but thoroughly unpleasant British film *Trainspotting*, in which one of the characters has himself locked in a room so that he might undergo withdrawal from the opiates he had been taking. If he had not been locked in the room, so the implication was, his symptoms would have been so severe he could not have tolerated them, and he would have been irresistibly obliged to seek drugs on the street; or he would have been driven to a mad, desperate and dangerous act. This scene was, from the point of view of a clinician who has personally observed hundreds of addicts withdrawing from opiates, so gross an exaggeration that it amounted to a travesty, probably deliberate; certainly, it served to reinforce the false view that the withdrawal effects of opiate addiction are almost too frightful to be contemplated. Actually, they are like flu – at their worst. Most addicts have few or no withdrawal effects at all.

There are further reasons why a phenomenon like withdrawal should be exaggerated, not only by the addicts themselves, but by society at large. Addicts thereby become compassion fodder, first for the intelligentsia, whose *raison d'être* is largely the search for people to pity, and second for an ever-increasing professional group that depends for its living, mortgage repayments and entire professional existence upon a category of victims, namely drug addicts. The workers in drug addiction clinics are at least as addicted to illicit drugs as are the addicts themselves, and the withdrawal effects would be vastly more painful for them and long lasting.

Hence the drug addict is turned into a victim for another reason, for only thus can he rightly be considered worthy of help and compassion. This is a modern form of bullying sentimentality, far cruder than that of our Victorian forebears. They divided the poor into the deserving and the undeserving, a division for which there is at least some justification; we divide everyone into victims and perpetrators. Only the former (by far the majority) are worthy of sympathy; the latter deserve only hatred. So if we are to extend sympathy to drug addicts, and therefore consent to help them, we must accord them victim status: that is to say, deny them responsibility for what they are or have become.

The equation of victimhood with desert of sympathy is, of course, sentimentalising nonsense, but it does explain why people must never be seen as the authors (even in part) of their own downfall. A recent court decision in the United States awarded a huge sum of money to a woman in her forties who had contracted lung cancer after smoking cigarettes for many years, on the grounds that the addictive properties of nicotine were not advertised at the time she took up smoking: though all sensible people already knew perfectly well that many smokers experienced difficulties in giving up (had not Mark Twain said that giving up smoking was the easiest thing to do in the world, because he'd done it hundreds of times?), and the harm that smoking does was by then already so well publicised that even people who knew little else knew that smoking was bad for them. The court chose to treat the woman as though she were the helpless victim of circumstance and manipulation by the tobacco companies – from which the lawyers want to extract endless compensation without actually driving them into bankruptcy, thus transferring the profits of the tobacco business from the shareholders to themselves, a form of larceny by litigation. If ever there were a case of sentimental infantilisation, in order to confer benefits upon someone to which they would not otherwise be entitled, this was it.

The young woman undoubtedly brought her lung cancer on herself. She knew what she was doing when she first started to smoke, and in all probability she did it in defiance of her parents' wishes and her school's rules. She knew that smoking was bad for her health, but chose to disregard her own knowledge, because the harmful effects of smoking were long distant, and the pleasures of smoking, and the kudos of defying the wishes of others as an assertion of her own independence of mind, were immediate. She could have abandoned the habit at any time in her smoking career, as millions of ex-smokers have proved, but she chose not to do so. To deny these obvious truths is to confer on her the doubtfully flattering status of automaton, without will or consciousness. And when finally disaster struck, she chose to blame others in the hope of monetary gain.

Does any of this mean that the doctors treating her lung cancer, insofar as it can be treated, should not accord her sympathy, should not attempt to alleviate her distress, should deny her painkillers when she has pain, should not procure for her as easeful a death as they are able? Should her doctors treat her anxiety about the children she would leave behind her with indifference or contempt, simply because she brought the situation upon herself? If sympathy and understanding are due only to immaculate victims, to those who did nothing to cause their own misfortune, are we to deny them to people injured through carelessness or through playing dangerous sports, to those who have lived not wisely but too well, to those who failed properly to heed a warning, to those with bad habits, in short to at least nine-tenths of the people who seek the help and advice of a doctor? The answer must surely be no.

What, then, should the doctor tell the patient? Should he pass judgement on the patient's failings, or should he merely skate over them delicately? The doctor, after all, is there to cure his patient, not to judge him.

The question of truth-telling is a delicate one, as I have already suggested. The truth is not for all occasions. The situation has to be taken into account. A comparatively young woman dying of lung cancer does not have to be confronted with her own part in her premature demise because there is simply no point in doing so. It would add cruelly to her distress, without any compensating advantage. When, however, she goes to law on the basis of her self-deception, the truth must be told: for in demanding restitution, her self-deception affects other people. She is, in effect, demanding that the truth be told.

Many are the painful truths that the doctor should withhold from the patient: indeed, many are the painful truths we must all withhold, if life is to be tolerable at all. We do not want to emulate Pavel Morozov, the little boy in Russia who, in the early 1930s, denounced his own parents as kulaks, and was taken up as an example for children to follow by the propaganda apparatus of the Stalinist state. (Not surprisingly, little Pavlik was murdered by enraged villagers, so that the martyr's crown was added to his reputation for truthfulness.) When to tell the truth, when to expose untruth and when to keep silent is itself a matter of subtle judgement.

When a patient tells the doctor an untruth, or is patently in a state of self-deception, should the doctor collude with it, when the untruth or the self-deception is precisely what is harming the patient? If it is not true, for example, that addiction is an illness just like any other, should the doctor pretend that it is, just to avoid a confrontation with his patient? When a man says that he cannot help hitting his sexual partner, that he goes into a blank state in which he does not know what he is doing, and when the woman who is hit in this fashion accepts that his violence towards her is a form of epilepsy over which he has no control, should the doctor passively accept this explanation as if it were worthy of credence? Should the doctor expose his patient's lies, half-truths and self-deceptions?

If the doctor does not do so, he risks giving the patient the impression that he is suffering from a disease like any other: that undesirable behaviour is a disease that he will cure by normal medical means. But since there is no such cure, and there is never likely to be such a cure, he is thereby deceiving the patient – who, of course, wants to be deceived, to gain 'official' confirmation of his own self-delusory beliefs. By failing to tell the patient the truth, the doctor is in fact prolonging the problem that the patient is asking him to solve. (If, by the way, my negative prediction that no medication will ever be developed that will prevent a patient who drinks too much from ever drinking again, or a drug addict from ever taking a drug again were to prove empirically false, I would willingly prescribe the miraculous agent, despite the fact that it would have overturned my whole philosophy and thereby injured my pride. The good of the patient is more important than my intellectual *amour propre*.)

Does the doctor's acknowledgement of the patient's responsibility for his own unhappy state mean, then, that he should not attempt to help the patient who indulges in self-destructive behaviour? By no means: there but for the grace of God goes he (doctors are themselves notoriously prone to suicide, alcoholism and drug addiction). His role in such cases is half medical, half pastoral. It is half medical because self-destructive habits have genuinely medical consequences, which only a doctor is in a position to understand; it is half pastoral because the self-destructive behaviour is not in itself a medical problem, but a psychological and moral one. In modern society, only a doctor is remotely able to tackle all these aspects at once. His task in the circumstances is to enable his patient to achieve self-knowledge through a form of Socratic dialogue.

Self-knowledge emphatically does not mean an endless trawl through the details of a patient's biography, looking for the buried psychological treasure whose uncovering will, in and of itself, solve the problem. This expectation, which is extremely widespread, is part of the baleful long-term cultural effect of psychoanalysis. A rumour has pervaded the world to the effect that Professor Freud used to rid unhappy young ladies of their paralysed limbs, and disturbed young men of their various perversions, by means of uncovering the psychic trauma that gave rise to them in the first place. Of course, the task of uncovering the trauma was in itself onerous, uncertain, difficult and lengthy; but once it was done, hey presto! – the problem was gone, like a magician's rabbit out of a hat. So when a man who drinks too much questions why he does so, he does not want a disquisition on the various factors that might be adduced, such as a genetic propensity or the fact that the time needed to earn the price of a bottle of whisky has halved, and therefore the number of people who drink to excess, among whom he is now one, has doubled. On the contrary, he wants the doctor to say, after many hours of intensive investigation (for no one likes the heart of his mystery to be plucked out too quickly), 'You drink because your mother did not hug you enough at the age of three.'

It might be asked how the doctor knows that this is the real, the true reason his patient drinks too much. The answer is simple. It is the true reason because, once uncovered and exposed to the open air, as it were, it stops the patient from ever drinking again. Similarly, if it fails to stop the patient from ever drinking again, the alleged true reason cannot be the real true reason. Therefore, the search must resume for the real true reason: a search that is liable to take many years, in the course of which the patient can continue to drink. His doctor, not he, has failed.

This is not to say, of course, that events do not affect people psychologically. It could hardly be otherwise with a creature endowed with both a conscious and an unconscious mind. The person who is violently robbed on the street is likely henceforth to be wary to the point of reclusion; a person who survives an air crash is likely to be nervous of flying again; those who have suffered an abusive childhood are unlikely to look upon the world as if the sun always shone and the birds always sung. But those who demand a biographical genesis of their own faults and disgruntlements are, at least in logic, believers in the doctrine of Original Sin. If their weaknesses are attributable to the misdeeds of others (and few who search their pasts for the liberating buried treasure are interested in the wrong decisions they have taken, usually often and usually in the joyous knowledge even at the time that they were wrong), then surely the misdeeds of others are themselves attributable to the misdeeds of yet others before them: and so on and so forth until we reach Adam and Eve. But in practice, no seeker of the buried treasure extends this explanatory method to the conduct of others: so that while he is content to regard his own behaviour as being conditioned by circumstances, he views the conduct of others with regard to him as being motivated by the purest malice, those others being fully autonomous human beings with unconditioned wills of their own. In short, he is not so much looking for an explanation as looking for an excuse.

While the doctor is not usually called upon to pass judgement upon his patients – he does not ask himself whether his patient with pneumonia makes a useful contribution to the world before he decides to treat him for it – the expansion of medicine into fields that were once hardly regarded as medical at all requires of the doctor more than a lazy adherence to the doctrine of never passing a judgement, especially when he is asked by his patient for advice. If a man comes to him complaining of unhappiness, and the doctor does not want to take the purist line that he is a doctor, not a pastor, he must try to ascertain, as far as is within his power, the cause of his patient's unhappiness. In fact, no such purist line is possible, since many of his patients will come to him complaining of symptoms that have no discernible pathological origin, but take their being from the unhappiness of the patient's life. And, as we have seen, bad habits often have dire medical consequences. Attention to his patient's soul (for lack of a better word) is inevitably part of the doctor's task: though there are some specialities, for example pathology, in which this aspect of the profession is much reduced.

Attention to a patient's soul can hardly be offered without a moral standpoint. In fact, though much effort has been expended by twentieth-century intellectuals to create a world in which there are no moral values except those of freedom and tolerance, it is actually impossible for human life to be lived without a much more detailed scale of values. It is almost as if Man were biologically primed to think in moral terms, in much the same way as he is primed to develop language. It is not so much that we do think morally as we must think morally: it is actually impossible to empty the human world of values and replace them purely with facts. In other words, when a man claims to be acting non-judgementally, not only is he making a judgement that it is better to be non-judgemental than judgemental (usually with a strong dose of self-congratulation into the bargain), but he is in effect replacing one set of values with another.

The loosening of the code in sexual matters, for example, is not the abandonment of morality: it is the acceptance of another code of morality. Clearly in many cases the doctor suspends moral judgement: the venereologist is not a preacher on behalf of moderation or faithfulness, let alone of chastity.

He is the healer of the pox, wherever he can be. But the doctor who treats the unhappiness, say, of the alcoholic cannot help, if he is serious, but delve into matters that are inextricably moral in nature. They cannot even be thought of, let alone improved, without moral categories.

Self-pity and self-deception are the great enemies of Mankind (of course, it is far easier to see them in others than to expunge them from one's own mind). The vicious cycle in which many alcoholics – and others with such compulsive habits – have entered goes as follows: I drink to forget my problems, my problems keep getting worse whatever I do, so I drink even more to forget them. The burden of the alcoholic's complaint is that the world has maltreated him. He does not consider that he has maltreated the world.

Last week, for example, a woman who drank too much and suffered certain medical consequences came to me. She drank first thing in the morning, and she drank last thing at night. Often she forgot what had happened the day before. She told me that she drank to forget her debts: she was being dunned for money by her creditors.

'How much do you owe?' I asked her.

'Five thousand pounds,' she replied.

'Accumulated over how long a period?'

'Years,' she replied.

'How many?'

'At least five.'

It was not difficult to demonstrate to her that during that period she had consumed vastly more than £5,000 worth of alcohol. Her tipple, she said, was Rémy Martin brandy, which costs £20 a bottle when drunk in the home and three times as much when drunk in the pub (as was her habit). On her own admission, she drank at least a bottle a day, and sometimes more, never missing a day. That is to say, on a very conservative estimate, she had, during the period of the accumulation of her debts, drunk £36,500 worth of brandy, seven times as much as her debt. In fact, she had probably drunk something like ten or fifteen times as much as her debts. She could easily have paid her debts and remained a very heavy drinker. It followed that she did not drink because of her debts; she did not start because of her debts, and she did not continue because of her debts. Her drinking had simply nothing to do with her debts, though when she told me that it had, she gave every appearance of believing what she said. To undeceive her was a necessary task if she were to change.

Of course, there may come a time when change is no longer possible or desirable. An alcoholic in his sixties, who has slid down the social scale, who has alienated his family to the point that no member of it will have anything further to do with him, who has no financial resources, who for many years has had no interests other than where the next bottle is coming from and the drunken banter of his drinking companions, and who is completely dependent upon handouts from the state, is not only unlikely to change, but has very little incentive to do so. If he were finally to give up drinking, what would his life be, in what respect would it improve? Could one recommend that he take up basket-weaving, or learn Sanskrit? Indeed, it is possible that sobriety and the clear-headedness that goes with it would destroy whatever remaining value he saw in life. Drunk, he would be able to tell himself that it was life that had abused him; sober, he would have to acknowledge that it was he who had abused life. And since this atrocious realisation would be uncompensated for by any possible improvement or restitution, it would be entirely pointless, unless knowledge of truth were a value that transcended all other values. This cannot be the view of the humane doctor.

To be a realist, then, the doctor must be a moralist, but not a moralist on all occasions. He must not be a moralising moralist, a kind of medical Southern Baptist teacher. He must judge delicately when and to what degree to introduce moral considerations into the consultation. He must have an idea in his mind of the relative weights of the technical and pastoral aspects of his task in any given consultation. He should not pass off moral problems as metabolic or pharmacological ones (or, of course, vice versa).

His morality must be a fairly elementary and uncontroversial one: that, for example, cruelty to and neglect of others is wrong. It is the duty of everyone to foresee and to weigh up, as far as is humanly possible, the consequences of his own actions. It is wrong wilfully to bring about circumstances in which others will suffer. It is right to learn from experience. It is necessary to review one's own life in order to do so, not to find excuses and to blame others (blameworthy as others might be). One is responsible for one's own actions and choices, and for the consequences that naturally result from these. Except in certain circumstances, one is not only a victim, even when one is a victim. It follows that a human being is never completely absolved of his responsibility: which is tiring, no doubt, and something from which we all want to escape now and again, but which at least also offers the hope that our fate is rarely completely out of our hands.

At first sight, it might seem wrong – against the all-forgiving, omnicompassionate ethic of Moses Maimonides – to speak to patients in this way, to make them face up to the responsibilities they would rather avoid. And of course it can be. You don't tell a dying person what a swine he's been all his life, and how he was hated by everyone who knew him because of his own intolerable behaviour. What is demanded or expected of a young adult is not reasonably demanded or expected of a pre-school child. The schizophrenic is absolved of responsibility for some of his acts or omissions (though it is interesting to note that the increase in violence committed by schizophrenics in society parallels pretty closely that committed by non-schizophrenics, suggesting that they are not completely out of touch with modern life). In general, we live in a climate of opinion in which it is easier to under- than to overestimate the degree of a person's responsibility.

It might be thought that, when a doctor attributes responsibility – either partial or whole – to a patient for his own unhappy situation, the patient would react with vehement denial and outrage that the doctor should dare to pass such judgement upon him. This has not been my experience – far from it. On the contrary, the patient has generally reacted with relief, as though the burden of living a lie has been lifted from his shoulders. There is no more difficult task than to go through life playing a part that never allows the mask to slip; and the distinction between self-deception and outright delusion is that there is a small, still voice in the mind of the self-deceived that tells him that he is telling lies, not only to others but to himself. There are far more self-deceived people in the world than deluded ones.

Of course, the doctor must exercise judgement in undeceiving the self-deceived. Self-deceit can be so strong that it resists all would-be undeceivers. It is not a question of intelligence, except insofar as the intelligent are able to produce more rationalisations more quickly and more effectively than the unintelligent. A patient of mine, a highly intelligent man, believed with all the vehemence of outraged righteousness that he had been unjustly and wrongfully imprisoned after he had physically attacked a witness in the witness box, in front of judge and jury: and not only that he was wrongfully imprisoned, but that he had contributed nothing whatever to his fate. There are some people whose undeceiving might cause them to kill themselves. There are others, increasingly numerous, who might become violent. The doctor must feel his way carefully, but without fear.

But most patients are pleased that the doctor accords them the respect that is due a fully conscious being, even one that has made innumerable and grievous mistakes. He does not adopt that unctuous, syrupy to-know-all-is-to-forgive-all manner that so often sounds like someone talking while straining at stool, a mixture of pain and prurient pleasure. His face is open and straightforward, rather than that of a man who is taking the weight of the world's woes upon his shoulders, for the time being at least. He accepts the patient as his moral equal by judging him by the same standards as he judges others: and the patient is no longer reduced to the expedient of playing victim as Marie Antoinette played shepherdess.

In order to do this, however, the doctor must recognise the limits of medicine, or of technicality. This requires judgement, because the limits are not like an iron curtain, with border guards to remind the wayward traveller. Indeed, the limits fluctuate, and it can never be quite certain where they are. But that there will always be such limits is certain: and just because there is a continuous spectrum does not mean we cannot truly distinguish between red and violet.

The patient often tells the doctor, for example, that he is suffering from a lack of self-esteem. Anyone who even considers the question of his self-esteem is, of course, lost: lost in a labyrinth of self-absorption that paradoxically excludes true self-examination. The patient who talks of his self-esteem is, in fact, asking the doctor to give him it: and such patients are growing in number. It is as if the doctor could pin self-esteem to someone's breast like a head of state decorating a brave soldier. But insofar as the concept of self-esteem has any worth at all, it is clear that it is a moral quality. This is proved by the fact that it is as bad to have too much as too little, as anyone who has seen the appalling swagger of young criminals in prison, many of whom have done terrible things to others, will attest. (Of course, some people might argue that the swagger of young criminals is a form of whistling in the wind, an outward overcompensation for the deep, and usually fully justified, lack of worth they feel within. If there is anything in this argument, the person who claims to feel a lack of self-esteem is, underneath it all, actually a raging egomaniac – a possibility that is certainly worth investigating.) Self-esteem is now regarded as a right, a little like social security payments. It is a manifestation of the philosophy of the Real Me: outwardly I may be a swine, perhaps I am a thorough nuisance to others, maybe I have never performed a good act in my life, it is possible that I am invariably selfish to all appearances, but deep inside, where the Real Me resides, there is a valuable person trying to get out, but he cannot for lack of self-esteem. The doctor is, of course, invited to go along with this charade, without alluding to his patient's bad qualities. But it would be better for him to encourage the patient's self-respect – an outward, other-regarding, unselfish social quality – than to join in sifting the tea leaves of his patient's deliberate evasions.

The failure to recognise limits – either where they are or even that there are any – explains a curious paradox: that, as the apparatus of care and concern grows ever more bloated, as more antidepressants than ever are swallowed, as therapies multiply like germs on a Petri dish, as life in short becomes ever more a search for therapy to heal the wounds, or the alleged wounds, within, there is no sign of a diminution of either misery or discontent: quite the contrary. My colleague, Dr Colin Brewer, put it wittily and succinctly: misery expands to meet the means available for its alleviation. In fact, one could put it even more strongly: misery always runs ahead of the means available for its alleviation.

The auguries are not good. In a secular age, people have no one but the doctor to turn to. Daily reports of scientific miracles encourage them to believe that 'there must be something' the doctor can do: the something being not the enunciation of the truth that will set them free, but a pill or an operation or a technique. And if something can be done, it follows that it ought to be done. The patient will henceforth live in a fever of enraged disappointment.

The doctor, for his part, believing that it is his duty and vocation always to bring succour, is likewise unwilling to believe that there is nothing he can do, at least by technical means, for his patient. He is also afraid of his patient's wrath. He is sucked into playing a part.

Medicine can cure some diseases, it can ease pain, it can bring comfort. But it will never alter the human condition, or relieve men of their responsibility.

Index